The Challenge for Primary Care

Nigel Starey

Director

Centre for Primary Care

University of Derby

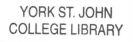
Foreword by

David Colin-Thome

General Practitioner

National Clinical Director of Primary Care

Department of Health

Radcliffe Medical Press

York St. John College

Radcliffe Medical Press Ltd
18 Marcham Road
Abingdon
Oxon OX14 1AA
United Kingdom

www.radcliffe-oxford.com
The Radcliffe Medical Press electronic catalogue and online ordering facility.
Direct sales to anywhere in the world.

British Library Cataloguing in Publication Data

A catalogue record for this book is available from the British Library.

ISBN 1 85775 569 3

Typeset by Advance Typesetting Ltd, Oxfordshire
Printed and bound by TJ International Ltd, Padstow, Cornwall

Contents

Foreword

Primary care in all its facets is central to the continuing success of the NHS. General practice is the most popular service, and research demonstrates it is also key to improving health outcomes. Despite what doubters may say, GPs and all the other primary care professionals are well regarded by the Department of Health, including those who work in NHS Direct and in the few Walk-In Centres, as all of us are essential in ensuring a responsive, quality service. Of fundamental importance are primary care trusts as funders of the local NHS and who are uniquely and heavily influenced by primary care clinicians.

As this is the policy context, my enjoyment of this book was even more enhanced. It is comprehensive in its coverage and explores the problematic and contentious issues in primary care and, indeed, the NHS at large. The prose is interspersed with the author's comments and views, many with which we would disagree. But to be challenged, informed and entertained is the hallmark of good communication. I feel this book achieves such laudatory aims and I recommend it.

David Colin-Thome
General Practitioner, Runcorn
National Clinical Director, Department of Health
and Visiting Professor, University of Manchester
March 2003

About the author

Primary care has always been a major part of Nigel Starey's life. He was brought up in rural Buckinghamshire where his first job was making pill boxes and bandaging leg ulcers for his father – a dispensing general practitioner (GP). After a first degree in biology and human genetics, Nigel studied medicine in London.

After training as a GP he was a partner in a rural dispensing practice in Burnham on Crouch for 10 years. He became a GP trainer and led the practice into first-wave GP fundholding. As a full-time GP, before the days of GP out-of-hours co-operatives, operating a strict personal list system and leading the development of fundholding in the area, Nigel became aware of the tensions and frustrations inherent in the system, and interested in the broader development of the primary care sector. Nigel spent three years working for North West Anglia Health Authority, as their medical advisor where he was involved with managing the relationships between general practice and NHS management – prescribing, emergency admissions, fundholding and service development, but also contributing locally and nationally to the development of a primary care-led health service. After three years, Nigel returned to general practice in Derbyshire, where, as part of a personal medical services (PMS) pilot project, he is involved with daily clinical care and is also a board member with the local primary care trust, with lead responsibility for clinical governance and cancer.

Nigel also directs the Centre for Primary Care at the University of Derby, where he teaches the double core module of the master's degree in primary care studies to students from a range of backgrounds from all over the world. Nigel is working with the HQS, CHIA and the GMC to implement their programmes in primary care. In addition, his interest in genetics has led him to work nationally to prepare the primary care sector for its emerging responsibilities in this area.

He has written and talked widely about the development of the British primary care sector and has particular interests in genetics, systems thinking, scenario planning, quality assurance and sustainable development.

Married with four children, Nigel lives on a small farm near Ashbourne, where he tries to interpret concepts of sustainability within a modern busy family and professional life.

Introduction

This book aims to help you, the reader, to understand the *'challenge'* that primary care within the United Kingdom's National Health Service (NHS) is facing, and the *'challenge'* it poses to the rest of the country's health and welfare system. Many of the issues have relevance in other countries and in systems beyond healthcare.

The past, present and future of the primary care system is an important area to analyse and critically evaluate, as it:

- plays a key role in the government's plans for modernising healthcare
- helps many individuals – from a range of backgrounds – who are now developing their careers within the sector and wish to contribute to the sector's success, fulfil their own ambitions and improve the quality of patient care.

So as to *understand, analyse* and *critically evaluate* the primary care sector, we shall explore it as both a *learning* system and an *evolving* system. Using two *caricatures* – sketches of alternative primary care futures – we shall look at the opportunities the sector has for further development and the risks and threats for all the parties. This is to help those involved with developing and planning the sector to understand its culture and its potential, so they can make wiser decisions about its future.

In order to understand, analyse and critically evaluate any system it is necessary to explore the following aspects.

- *How it has developed* – its heritage, its responsibilities, the values, attitudes and beliefs of those who work within the sector and the value of the heritage to the wider public services.
- *The elements making up the system.* As part of our education we are taught to analyse problems by breaking them down into their constituent parts – it makes it simpler to understand each element if we can look at it on its own. The only problem is that if we take a machine to pieces completely and understand each element, it may be very difficult to put it back together again. Anyone who has ever taken a car engine or a sewing machine to pieces will understand the difficulties. Nevertheless, it does make it easier to understand the whole system if we have some appreciation of its constituent parts.
- *Synthesising the elements.* If we are to understand the primary care system we need to appreciate that each of the elements plays a part in the workings of the whole system. We need to understand the inter-relationship of the elements and the part that each plays in maximising the efficiency and effectiveness of the whole. We will look at a number of ways of understanding how the primary care system works so that we have not just an appreciation of the laws or rules governing its behaviour, but also sufficient understanding to be able

to analyse problems that arise and attempt to devise reasonable solutions to them.

- *What fuels the system?* It is all very well to take an engine to pieces, understand how the elements work, put it back together again, see how all the elements interact with each other and what the purpose of each element is, etc., but we also need to understand what powers the engine. Any system requires energy or resources to drive it and the primary care system is no different. As well as requiring energy as an input, the system will also produce energy as an output. While a car engine turns petrol into the force to make the car travel down the road, the primary care system uses human resources and money to provide care for the population.

Understanding its heritage and analysing the primary care system can help us to interpret how fit the system is for its current and developing responsibilities. Using the tools of systems thinking – analysing the whole primary care system, how it fits together, how it operates, how it responds and how it cares – requires us to understand a little bit about *systems thinking* itself. This should equip us to see not only the *wood for the trees*, but also the *wood and the trees*.

Having considered the design of the primary care system, and its heritage, looked in some detail at how fit the system is for its current and emerging responsibilities, the next step is to consider how those responsibilities might develop over future years. Although the future is always a little unpredictable, we have to make plans for it. The best plans are based on an understanding of how things have happened in the past, an appreciation of the trends that might be expected to continue into the future, and an understanding of the forces that are driving the present into the future. We shall use two examples to help us tease out some of these trends and forces.

This book attempts to equip you, the reader, with an understanding of the primary care sector which is sufficient to help you be a *master* of it. Mastering a subject requires a level of understanding which goes beyond that required of an amateur dabbling in the subject and beyond that required of a practitioner practising the subject.

Whether you are a professional practitioner in the primary care system, a non-executive director of a new corporate organisation governing the primary care sector, a student of health policy or a patient, you will already have a wealth of relevant knowledge and experience which will help you to master this subject.

After 50 years of the NHS we are entering the twenty-first century facing major challenges. The complexity and costs of modern health services and the dynamics of the society for which those services are provided have changed radically since the early post-war years when the NHS was born. The design of the system, which might have been fit for the purpose in 1947, is now being redesigned to be fit for the twenty-first century. While UK general practice may still use 'Lloyd George' envelopes and rely on an organisational form

– *professional partnership* – which have served it well thus far, it may not equip it, and the rest of the primary care sector, to adapt to its emerging responsibilities. As new technology allows more and more care to be provided outside hospital, as the population ages, and as everyone's aspirations for perfect health increase, so the responsibilities of the primary care sector have expanded and will continue to expand. If a greater proportion of healthcare is to be provided outside hospital, then a greater proportion of NHS resources will be spent there. Inevitably the primary care sector will be held to account for the quality of care that it provides and for its effective use of resources. The changing dynamics of the whole healthcare system as a result of primary care having the responsibility to *commission* hospital care, *assess* the health needs of the local community and work in *partnership* with social services, also means that it has a broader range of responsibilities to account for.

In addition to the above considerations concerning the operation of the primary care system and how it is evolving to meet its emerging responsibilities, we also need to reflect on the dynamism of the system's relationship with other parts of the economy. There is little point in mastering the primary care system without understanding how it interacts with:

- the social security and pension system
- the voluntary sector
- the education system
- the commercial sector and, in particular, the pharmaceutical industry
- local government, including social services, housing, environmental health and planning.

If the primary care sector is to work in partnership with the organisations represented in each of these bullet points, then we need to understand what partnership working involves, the purpose of the partnerships and the differing interests that each partner will have.

We cannot allow the concept of 'partnership' to be a rather vague, ill-defined solution to all the system's problems – analysing *partnership* should help us find a range of organisational arrangements which suit particular circumstances. On the whole, relationships and systems work the way they do because that is how they are designed, how the elements fit together best and how they work together most comfortably.

This then is the agenda. The book does not seek to impart facts, but rather to help readers construct, analyse and criticise; above all this book is offered as an aid and stimulus to your own thinking.

CHAPTER 1

The heritage

Introduction

The well-developed primary care sector in the United Kingdom is not an accident of history. Barbara Starfield points out[1] that strong development of a primary care sector is often associated with a more efficient and effective healthcare system overall. To understand why the UK primary care sector has evolved the way it has, and indeed why it is currently taking on an even more powerful position as controller of resource allocation across the whole health service, we need to look at the context within which the sector has developed, the forces which have moulded its services and its designers, who have left such a rich heritage behind them. If we are to understand how the sector may evolve and change in future, then we need to appreciate how it has evolved thus far and why it behaves the way it does. This chapter explores the development of some of the elements making up the primary care sector in the United Kingdom so as to provide an historical context to later chapters.

Society in the United Kingdom has changed dramatically during the twentieth century. Following the *industrial* revolution and social turmoil of the nineteenth century, the twentieth century produced a *social* revolution. The emancipation of women following the First World War is only one example of a major trend which saw the rise of organised labour, emancipation of men and women through universal education, and redistribution of wealth – all leading to the blurring and gradual disappearance of the British class system. This social revolution has fundamentally shaken and changed the values and beliefs that underpinned Victorian society and is, of course, reflected in similar social revolutions in other countries. Even in Victorian times, health services in the United Kingdom were made up of a partnership between private enterprise, the voluntary sector, and public provision. The heritage of Victorian hospitals is a testament to both this public provision and the charitable and voluntary sector, which left us with many of our great teaching institutions as well as endowed wards, beds and cots. The Red Cross, St John Ambulance Association and the tradition of a strong community nursing profession reflect this heritage of community healthcare.

Primary care services at the beginning of the twentieth century were less organised and less developed than services in the hospital sector. Isolated single-handed medical practitioners, apothecaries, dentists and pharmacists were not universally available to the whole population whose access to health services depended primarily on their ability to pay, where they lived and their class. The Victorian heritage of 'the market' meant that it was economic forces that determined an individual's health and the population's health status.

The social revolution of the twentieth century has included a revolution in the primary care sector, which has responded to, and been the result of, the forces unleashed by the revolution elsewhere. In society at large the rapid pace of change throughout the twentieth century, and indeed the increasingly rapid change in the last decades of the century, has inevitably challenged the ability of health services to respond and evolve as rapidly. Individuals, professional groups and organisations only change when they have to (Napoleon realised this) and, rather than rush into it enthusiastically, most have to be coerced to change. Such has been the experience of the revolution in the primary care sector, but just as King Canute could not halt the tides by 'royal command', so you cannot halt the social revolution by individual or professional dictate.

The designers

The employed workforce received primary medical care under Lloyd George's National Insurance Act of 1911, but their wives and families had to pay.[2] In his 1918 Cavendish lecture, Bertrand Dawson, a physician from the London Hospital and a wartime military doctor, described how a comprehensive health service could be co-ordinated. In 1920, he was invited to chair a consultative council on the future provision of health services and was the first to propose a hierarchical system of primary care centres linked to district hospitals and regional centres linked to university teaching hospitals.[3,4] Although largely a professionally dominated model based on a purely medical 'disease management' view of healthcare provision, this early design left us with two important elements which are still discernible in the British primary care sector today.

1   First the idea of registration and a lifelong medical record resulted from the Lloyd George reforms and indeed many general practices still use the traditional Lloyd George envelope, which, at least in theory, contains the lifelong medical record of every registered patient.
2   Second, Dawson recognised that treatment services on their own would be insufficient to ensure the health of the population. The need for health promotion and disease prevention services was highlighted and has become an increasingly important part of modern primary care provision. The importance of immunisation to control infectious disease and of health promotion to counteract the harmful effect of social behaviour, such as smoking, alcohol and drug abuse, are examples of this.

In addition to Lloyd George's National Insurance Act and the medical leadership provided by Lord Dawson, the inter-war years saw some experimentation into the development of primary healthcare teams, such as those linked to urban regeneration schemes in Aberdeen and south London. Increasingly close links between medical practice and nursing in the community were developing through local nursing associations and their links with hospital practice, local authority services and general practice.

Although 'vocation' was an important part of the ethos of both nursing and medical practice in the community between the wars, there were important differences in their approach. Medicine had to make a profit if doctors were to live and this involved competition for patient registrations as well as private practice. Nursing was salaried; nurses were employed and managed to the extent that they were less driven by money than by the process and operational detail of individual care. Thus, primary care medicine developed as small *private* sector businesses in isolation from *community* nursing, but shared some of the values of commitment to local individuals and communities. Their different social standing and employment conditions led to tensions in their working relationships, which still exist today. Similarly, working relationships with other members of the modern primary healthcare team, e.g. community pharmacists, counsellors, physiotherapists, occupational therapists, dieticians, chiropodists, speech therapists, etc., are relatively young and reflect similar tensions to those described above. Many have their roots in hospital practice or local authority community services, rather than as part of a general medical practice. In the case of community pharmacy, the tensions between doctors who dispense – as most did between the wars – and pharmacists who supply continue to the present day because of the dispensing doctor regulations.

Box 1.1: Joyce's story

Joyce is, and has always been, a community nurse. After qualifying at St Mary's Paddington she trained as a midwife, health visitor and district nurse before moving to the Chilterns in 1939. Employed by the county nursing association, she was responsible for the nursing care of a scattered rural community in an area of 100 square miles. She lived in a tied house, drove an Austin Seven provided for her, had few holidays and little time off. She lived frugally, but was respected and cherished by the local community – free nursing care was available to everyone, even if the doctor had to be paid.

Joyce worked closely with Dr Elliott, the local general practitioner, who lived in a large house with an attached consulting room and dispensary. They frequently used their complementary skills in partnership; they respected and supported each other – but they did not often mix socially, did not consult together and were quite clear that 'doctor's orders' were what drove the system.

Early in the Second World War Dr Elliott had a stroke and became less mobile. There was no other medical care available, so Joyce spent much of her time acting as his eyes and ears – doing nearly all the home visiting, acting as his driver and confidant – and developing a healthy respect for his judgement. Three hundred home deliveries were carried out with virtually no medical back-up available as the flying squad in Oxford was over two hours away. Chronic and acute disease, such as TB, cancer, osteomyelitis and sepsis, were dealt with before antibiotics, childhood fevers before immunisation and pregnancy without scans or rhesus testing.

Following the war, things gradually improved with the arrival of the NHS, more medical and nursing staff, the telephone and television. In the 1960s Joyce got married. She had to give up her pension rights, nurse's bungalow and car as they went with the job which was not a married person's post. When she retired she was fêted by the community she had given so much of her life to – parties and presents, but no pension.

Twenty years later, widowed and not in the best of health, Joyce is now living in a private care home. Her cottage is for sale to help pay the fees. Her story is told alongside that of her recent experience in hospital – the noise, the delays, the fog of post-op confusion and the kindness of ancillary staff and old friends. There is no benevolence fund for Joyce, and she doesn't want charity; there is no home for retired nurses where she can be among her peers. There are only her wonderful memories, her experience and the love and respect of the community to fortify her.

The birth of the NHS

The 1942 Beveridge Report[5] proposed state funding for the nationalised health service and aimed for universal coverage to tackle 'five giants' on the road to reconstruction after the war:

- want
- disease
- ignorance
- squalor and
- idleness.[6]

This report, allied to the report of the British Medical Association's (BMA's) medical planning commission in 1942, which also called for a comprehensive service covering the population, made it possible for the post-war Labour government to introduce the National Health Service Act in 1948. The service was born into the post-war climate of austerity, crisis and shortages made worse by the harsh winter of 1947. The social revolution which had emancipated women and transformed the workforce, housing and education, now saw the provision of a National Health Service as an important social priority, alongside nationalisation of core industries and social security, education and housing reforms. Unlike other industrialised Western countries, whose experience of the social revolution in the twentieth century was different, the British 'socialist' approach served to marry the differing histories of the professions involved and the institutions and organisations that had previously provided healthcare.

As far as primary care services were concerned, they were seen as peripheral to the main thrust of the NHS Act, which served to develop and nationalise hospital and specialist services. GPs remained self-employed, independent contractors, but provided comprehensive general medical services to the whole population; nurses, midwives and health visitors became state employees; and pharmacists, opticians and dentists worked under similar national arrangements to general medical practitioners. Primary care services were funded partly from local authority funds, and partly from general medical service allocations from Parliament. The original Act emphasised the development of health centres,[7] which would be built, equipped and staffed at public expense and provide medical, dental and health promotion services plus associated specialist outpatient sessions. Unfortunately, lack of finance meant such centres were seldom provided. The 18 000 GPs, mostly male and over half of them working alone, usually practised from their own homes. Administrative and support staff were almost entirely lacking (apart from the doctor's wife) and facilities were often rudimentary. The Act introduced a Medical Practices Committee, which helped to redistribute GPs, over time, to areas with doctor shortages and to restrict access to areas with excess doctors.

A patient's guide produced by the Ministry of Health in 1948 said that as everyone could now have a GP, it was the GP who would: 'arrange for the patient every kind of specialist care he himself is unable to give. Except in emergencies, hospitals and specialists would not normally accept a patient for advice or treatment unless they had been sent by his family doctor.'[8] This ethos served to institutionalise the referral system and the gatekeeping role of the GP which, before the NHS, had been an ideal doctors aimed at. With the establishment of the NHS, gatekeeping served as an effective way of controlling patient demand and ensuring the protection of specialist services. The 'gatekeeper system' established the separation of primary and secondary care, with the referral letter and discharge note being the currency of transfer between the sectors. Family doctors defended the system because they had continuing responsibility for individual patients, consultants because it protected them from cases which might be trivial or outside their fields of interest and the government defended it because it saved money to have a filter in the system. The fundamental relationship between GP and specialist had been altered. Previously, specialists made most of their money from private practice and therefore courted GPs for referrals; after the establishment of the NHS, specialists had less need to court GPs for private work, but also had little reason to be grateful to them for deluging them with NHS referrals.

The dynamics

The birth of the NHS into the austere, resource constrained, battered and bruised post-war British society cannot be considered as an isolated event. Rather, the birth followed a long gestation:

- from the time of the industrial revolution and the gradual organisation of medical and nursing care
- from the forces released by the social revolution, which liberated the British people from:
    - the suppression of personal conscientiousness due to lifelong servitude
    - the exclusion of half the population from full participation in the affairs of the country until women's emancipation after the First World War
    - the distortions of the class system which affected access to education, health services and economic resources as well as power
    - the crisis of identity which crumbling British imperialism faced as a result of two world wars and their effect on the values of the nation.

The founding principles of the welfare state, outlined in the Beveridge Report, specified that the *nation* had a responsibility to its population *as a community* – a responsibility to invest during the good times to ensure that the weak, the sick, the elderly and the socially disadvantaged would be looked after in their time of need, implying an end to the exaggerations of market forces having free reign over welfare issues. While important in themselves, developments such as the NHS Act, the Dawson Report and the Beveridge Report were merely stages in the process of individual liberation and communal, social responsibility which the social revolution of the twentieth century released.

Of course, such energies can either be directed constructively or can conflict with each other to inhibit progress. In physiological processes, the individual elements of a system are linked together and are dependent on each other for success – similar principles apply in industrial systems, education, etc. All of these systems require energy and are controlled by a complex system of positive and negative feedback loops so that the efficiency and effectiveness of the system are maximised. Figure 1.1 illustrates the simplest kinds of feedback system; more complex ones such as those controlling fertility or blood pressure will be familiar to many.

In these terms, the birth of the NHS can be considered as the logical response, or intervention by the British community, to the forces released by the social revolution and the necessity to re-value the resources of the nation following

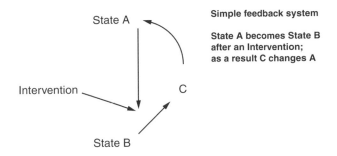

Figure 1.1: The simplest kind of feedback system.

the predations of war. In Figure 1.1 C is the consequence on society of the introduction of the NHS. As a result of the NHS, A becomes B. B feeds back and changes A, which, as a result of more feedback, changes B, etc. The result is a system of intervention, development and feedback. This is an evolving or dynamic system:

- responsive to the community's requirements
- sensitive to technological change and social forces
- constantly changing and evolving in response to circumstance.

Primary care 1950–95

The NHS Act (1946) translated the work of the earlier 'designers' of health services into a truly national system. For the first time the NHS gave the whole population the right of access, free at the point of use, to a general practitioner or family doctor. The unique position of the family doctor as the patient's advocate and as gatekeeper to the rest of the health and welfare service was designed in from the start. The doctor's role was to act both as an independent counterweight to a centralised, bureaucratic and impersonal service, and as a care co-ordinator controlling or regulating access to specialist services.

Universal registration through a national contract with highly centralised admin-istration was the process by which the national service was established, along with the associated redistribution of resources and clear definition of the patient's and practitioner's rights and responsibilities. A continuation of the registration cards originally introduced by Lloyd George (and in the author's experience still treasured by those who were entitled to them in the inter-war years) helped to symbolise the universal enfranchisement that the NHS introduced. General practice, and in particular general medical practitioners, by virtue of registration and gatekeeping, became the most powerful players in the primary sector at the birth of the NHS. Inevitably, in the sea of pathology that the NHS inherited, disease management rather than health promotion or the prevention of disease was the top priority and, therefore, the pre-eminence of the 'medical model' was entirely understandable. The pre-eminence of the medical model did, however, mean that primary care nursing, dentistry, ophthalmic services and the professions allied to medicine were only empowered 'second hand' and became dependent on the medical model for their influence. Patients were essentially 'supplicant', more dependent on the doctor's ethical behaviour than before, as they were no longer paying directly for his or her service.

An early report into the state of general practice was funded by the Nuffield Trust in 1948. Dr Joseph Collins surveyed a variety of English practices and found great variation in their standards. In city practices, he saw *no* examples of effective practice and described surgeries without any facilities for examination, without any systematic record keeping and without any facilities for proper consultation. The country doctor tended to know his patients better and to spend more time with them. Many GPs seemed to be competent and effective clinicians, but taken 'as a whole' the report was a damning indictment of the state of English general practice. There seemed to be no definition of quality of care and no standards against which to monitor performance. Collins noted that the worst practice tended to be found where the population's need was greatest and that good quality practice tended to be in areas furthest away from large hospitals. Some premises required condemnation in the public interest. Dr Collins recommended the establishment of primary care teams, linking doctors, nurses, social workers and technicians in group practices serving 15 000–25 000 people. He blamed the widening gap between hospital and primary care on a lack of political interest at local and national levels, and on the failure of the national contract and nationalised administration to invest in the development of primary care services.[9]

The Collins Report was followed by the BMA sponsored Hadfield Report[10] and the Taylor Report[11] on good general practice: 'in the final analysis, quality of the service depends on the men or women who are actually doing the job'.[11] The response to these early reports pointing out the weakness of the primary care sector was an increase in investment such as recommended by the Danckwerts Report,[12] which moved remuneration away from a flat capitation rate and introduced a basic practice allowance and financial encouragement for single-handed practitioners to form partnerships and group practices. A more even distribution of doctors was being encouraged by the Medical Practices Committee and there was a steady decrease of patients living in areas of doctor shortage through the early 1950s. The Royal College of General Practitioners (RCGP) was established so that family medicine, with its own skills and knowledge base, would have its own academic body, curriculum, research and college to promote it. As early as 1952, the minister, Ian McCloud,[13] called for investment in general practice in order to improve its status, be of benefit to patients and cut waiting lists. He encouraged the development of group practices and primary care teams, including midwives, district nurses and health visitors, and closer working with dentists, pharmacists and opticians. Thus the vision from the minister, the nascent RCGP and further investment began the renaissance of general practice in the mid- to late 1950s.

Taken together this represents an analysis of general practice as part of the primary care system and a description of how leverage and a framework of incentives could develop and change the system.

Towards the end of the 1950s and throughout the 1960s the development of training courses for GPs received more attention. The College of General Practitioners,[14] co-ordinated by John Horder, recommended two years' postgraduate education in supervised general practice and three years in hospital posts. He also recommended the establishment of academic departments for general practice in every medical school. These were the early moves to establish the discipline of general practice, but were restricted to general medical practice, rather than the broader remit of primary care services. This meant that the development of nursing and the other professions allied to medicine, along with pharmacy, dentistry, etc., received less consideration. Naturally, the development of new pharmaceutical products and the expansion of the pharmaceutical industry meant that dispensing pharmacy and the relationship between the industry and the NHS began to become more important. Advertising and pharmaceutical representatives focused on general practitioners as the 'prescribers'. This was the era of rapid expansion in the availability of new effective medicines – antibiotics, benzodiazepines, beta blockers, etc. all began to transform the range of medication available to general practitioners to manage their patients' pathologies effectively outside hospital.

So the evolution of primary care as a system meant looking at general practice development, but also at all the other elements in the system.

The 'pool system' through which general practitioners were paid did little to reward good practice and by the early 1960s a further review considering the future of family doctors was required. The essential feature of the pool system was that almost all payment was made from a national 'pool' without any consideration of:

- the health needs of local communities
- the range of services offered by practices
- the costs of providing them.

There was therefore little encouragement for practitioners to invest in developing better services for patients and little extra reward for providing better care.

Leverage – or an incentive framework – was needed to improve the quality of care patients received.

A further review, *The Field Work of the Family Doctor*,[15] looked ahead to what the family doctor was likely to be doing over the succeeding 10–15 years and served to lay the foundations for the development of general practice and the broader primary care sector. In it, Gillie saw the GP of the future as the co-ordinator of the resources of hospital and community care, i.e. the effective gatekeeper. Although not universally welcomed by all GPs, the Gillie Report formed the backdrop to negotiations with the Wilson government in 1964 when Kenneth Robinson, as Minister of Health, negotiated the 1966 GPs' charter with Dr James Cameron (General Medical Services Committee chairman). This charter, negotiated in difficult circumstances, turned the tide in general practice. The number of GPs recruited began to rise, investment in premises and in the development of primary care teams expanded, and incentives to improve the quality of care patients received were welcomed. There was an upsurge of interest in health centres, the development of GP training and postgraduate education through postgraduate centres, usually based in hospitals.

Although sometimes described as a seminal event, the 1966 charter can also be viewed simply as another turn of the evolutionary wheel – a step towards the dynamic, high quality, responsive system the community requires.

In 1962, the report of the BMA's Committee of Inquiry into the NHS – chaired by Sir Arthur Porritt – was published. It supported the continued development of the NHS as a state-funded monopoly, encouraging private practice in order to challenge the state monopoly's tendency to sloth and indolence and to protect professional freedom. The report supported the continuation of the tripartite funding arrangements (*see* above), but suggested that the services should be brought together under a single area board so that management across local authority, primary care and hospital sectors could be better co-ordinated. This report, alongside the Gillie Report,[15] prepared the ground for the development of the NHS for the next 10–15 years. The agreement between the GPs and the government, leading to the new GP contract in 1966, secured new funding for general practice, provided the infrastructure for the development of effective primary care teams supporting professional practice and improved services for patients. The move from single-handed practice to partnerships with the employment of administrative and secretarial support and practice nurses was promoted along with the move to purpose-built premises, continued professional development and some incentives to provide a broader range of health services to a smaller population through 'item of service fees' forming a larger proportion of income. Unfortunately, as with all negotiated solutions, there were some compromises in the charter. The financial arrangements, 'the pool', did not radically shift resources to tackle health problems and health inequalities, or to reward high quality innovative practice. In addition, the charter looked at general practice but was not matched by similar arrangements for other independent contractors, district nurses, health visitors or midwives. The charter did not look at the role of general practitioners working in hospitals and did not co-ordinate primary care, hospital care and local authority services. The role of general practice in promoting the health of the community (the public health role) similarly remained underdeveloped. General practice, the primary care team and the broader primary care workforce continued to focus on the management of disease, remained reactive to the demands of individual patients and remained relatively isolated from the rest of the health service. The administration of general practice and other independent contractors remained the responsibility of 'the executive committee' and was not integrated with the management of the rest of the health service as recommended by the Porritt Committee.

Because the development of the system has been 'stepped' rather than continuous – intervention, report, intervention, etc. – it has always been subject to interruption and manipulation as a result of economic or political pressures.

For many GPs, the years following the 1966 charter were regarded as a golden age of new investment, administrative support, better premises and better support for professional practice with training programmes and continuing professional development. Nevertheless, workload remained heavy and the relative professional isolation of practitioners meant variations in standards of care. In addition, the active questioning of the power of the medical profession and the paternalistic relationship between doctor and patient had begun. Illich[16] articulated and interpreted the risks involved to all sides, while access to television programmes fuelled public knowledge about health and demystified medicine. The economic constraints of the 1970s, with inflation, fuel crises and industrial disputes, affected the health service as much as any other sector of society so that while the 1966 charter introduced much needed investment and reform, general practice and the broader primary care sector were not free to grow and develop in isolation from the broader developments in society. In addition, technological change introduced new therapies enabling treatment at home, e.g. treatment for peptic ulcers and home dialysis, and shorter lengths of stay in hospitals. The process of de-institutionalisation began and has gone on to affect care of the elderly and mental health and learning disabilities care, as well as care in acute hospitals. These processes have changed the nature of primary healthcare and challenge many of the professional roles and responsibilities involved in the sector.

So technological and social changes and the forces they involve also affect the development cycle.

The late 1970s and early 1980s saw further reviews of general practice, with attempts to tackle the variation in quality and the emerging need to develop health promotion and disease prevention within primary care, as well as providing effective management of acute and chronic disease. Sadly, political posturing and the intransigence of GP negotiators inhibited progress. The lack of effective leadership to address the 'quality' and 'improving health' agendas meant that little progress was made in providing a more effective primary care sector to meet the needs of the population during the 1980s. The internal market, a new GP contract in 1990 and the introduction of GP fundholding brought new dynamism into the health service, challenging traditional planning models and introducing more responsiveness to local circumstances and market forces. Unfortunately, the issues of fairness and of responsiveness to the varying needs of individuals and populations were not adequately dealt with. The internal market and GP fundholding challenged many practitioners' views of social responsibility and the purpose of the health service and, in pure economic terms, the jury remained undecided about the benefits of the reforms until they were swept away by the election of the Labour government in 1997. Nevertheless, the legacy of the Conservative reforms of the 1990s in preparing the primary care sector for the challenges of the modern world should not be ignored:

- the moves towards corporacy
- the understanding of the need for more appropriate governing arrangements of the sector
- the need for teamworking and planning in primary care
- the changing relationship between consumers of healthcare and the professions providing that care.

These were all emerging themes through the 1990s and have been further developed in recent years.

In fundholding we see how a further intervention has consequent feedback effects on the primary care system – it is not an end in itself, merely another step towards ...

The last years of the Conservative administration saw the development of new initiatives such as total purchasing projects, out-of-hours GP co-operatives and whole district primary care projects such as in Wakefield. These presaged the development of new corporate primary care developments, which were to be piloted through the Primary Care Act of 1997. This approach to letting '1000 flowers bloom' through a process of experimentation, was transformed following the election of the Labour government which rapidly moved to end GP fundholding and introduced corporate organisations in primary care as described in the white paper,[17] *The New NHS: modern, dependable.* But they used many of the 'tools' and approaches of the previous administration – pilot projects, co-operatives, etc., did not end, they just evolved further.

Paralleling the development of general practice and medicine in primary care throughout the twentieth century have been developments in the other professions involved with primary care, which similarly have responded to changes in society and technology but whose heritage, culture and approaches to professionalism have distinct differences that continue to influence their development. A brief description of their development is important if readers are to appreciate how the current primary care sector is the product of its heritage and is having to harness that heritage to the changing agenda of the twenty-first century.

Box 1.2:   Eight issues for GPs

1   To swallow their pride and realise the power of teamworking across professional boundaries.
2   To loosen their control over those aspects of primary care which they are not best equipped to control, e.g. capital, employment, management, organisational development and therapy management.
3   To sharpen their focus on diagnosis, care planning and co-ordination so that their special skills in these areas are not overwhelmed.
4   To loosen their rigid career structure so that fulfilling and flexible options are available to all qualified practitioners.
5   To open up practice to external review, to embrace quality assurance and value the patient's experience.
6   To move further away from patronising paternalism and the dependency culture towards a professionalism characterised by expertise in diagnosis and medical practice alongside mutual respect for and trust of patients, colleagues and the wider population.
7   To end isolationism – to start working with hospital colleagues when patient care demands it, to let nurses, pharmacists and other care professionals take responsibility when they have the right skills and to give care back to patients and their families so that their autonomy is cherished.
8   To value themselves for their special skills and contribution – to free themselves from the burden imposed by the pedestal they have sat on, so that they can support and contribute rather than control and manipulate.

Nursing

The three branches of the nursing profession working in the community – district nursing, midwifery and health visiting, have long and honourable histories. While district nursing often remained the responsibility of the voluntary sector, with local district nursing associations funding the local service, health visiting has a history based in radical local politics and the development of community services by local authorities. The public health function of health visitors, preventing disease and promoting health through improved sanitation and personal behaviour, has long been part of the health visiting philosophy. Midwifery is really a separate profession from nursing, although many nurses take it up. Between the wars, the great majority of births took place in the home supervised by midwives who would call for medical intervention only if complications arose. Although in rural areas, nurses might be 'triple qualified', fulfilling midwifery, health visiting and district nursing functions, in most places the three nursing services operated separately and not always harmoniously. The working conditions of each service were determined by their employers and could be quite different. District nurses, for example, were often not permitted to marry and, if they did, they risked losing their home, their employment and their pension, while health visitors employed by local authorities enjoyed better working conditions.

Nursing in the community has developed informally as an extension of family care since the original Poor Laws in the time of Elizabeth I. More formally, outreach of religious orders during the early nineteenth century and then the establishment of district nursing in the 1850s reflected the changes in society at the time. The need for a healthier workforce, the Victorian virtue of charitable giving and voluntary effort, and the emerging relationship between free enterprise and individual responsibility were influential.

Just as pharmacy established itself as a profession separate from medicine during the nineteenth century's industrial revolution, with a separate educational, regulatory, ethical and organisational basis, so too did nursing.

From their early beginnings in the 1850s both district nursing and health visiting followed an employed model rather than a self-employed or small 'shopkeeper' model. Employment was with local authorities or voluntary nursing associations. Management of nursing was either through the medical officer of health or through senior nurses in the county nursing associations. The traditional role of district nursing is the provision of 'personal care'. Illness creates dependency: the sick need not only medical treatment involving diagnosis, therapy and monitoring until recovery but also personal service and personal care. The provision of these services and the administration of the treatment which the doctor prescribes, have been the two basic duties of the nurse. By her skilful care, the sick can be restored to health.[18]

Health visiting represents an extension to this role, as it has evolved to support the healthy rather than treat the sick. Fulfilling an executive public health function, health visitors from the 1850s have had an educational and advisory function in support of social change. Promoting healthy behaviour, tackling poor sanitation, etc. has meant that their knowledge base is much more about counselling and teaching than about practical nursing. Nevertheless, their effectiveness at tackling infant mortality, breastfeeding, immunisation and child protection is difficult to separate from the efforts of others and of wider social change.

Other branches of nursing have also evolved in response to the industrial and social revolutions. School nursing was first introduced during the Boer War as it was recognised that the health status of school children left much to be desired. Community psychiatric nursing has evolved largely as an outreach service from specialist mental health provision as a response to the changing pattern of care of people with psychiatric illness.

The establishment of a nursing register (1923), by the Royal College of Nursing, of formal education encompassing both theory and practice and the development of an appropriate career structure reflecting specialist interests and responsibilities has largely developed during the time of the NHS.

The emergence of nurses (practice nurses) employed by general practitioners during and since the 1970s added another dimension to nursing in primary care. These 'treatment room' nurses have helped move general practice from its traditional disease management focus to a more systematic approach to chronic disease management, disease prevention and health promotion. Nevertheless, the lack of an appropriate syllabus for education and development, any career structure and access to power in general practice has meant that practice nursing has attracted nurses whose ambition is more limited than those seeking advancement in a hierarchical, structured career such as district nursing or health visiting.

These different branches of primary care nursing, along with others such as community midwifery, specialist outreach provisions such as renal and cancer nursing and voluntary sector provisions such as Red Cross and Marie Curie nursing, make up a very heterogeneous primary care nursing profession. The idea that they are all nurses is often less strongly adhered to than in the medical profession. Rather, nurses identify more with the branch of the nursing profession to which they belong and give more loyalty to that branch. This fragmentation, which has been perpetuated through the different employment and career structures of the branches, is now being questioned by primary care trusts as they bring together general practice provision, community trust provision and social services provision with the voluntary sector to begin to plan provision of services which meet the health needs of their local community. Nurses are important members of the management boards of primary care trusts (PCTs) and the new responsibilities they have been assuming, such as nurse prescribing, nurse triage and nurse practitioner roles will have profound implications for the future of the nursing profession within the primary care sector.

In moving from a disease service to a health service, nursing is being transformed from a caring, personal service oriented profession. Where it is going is less clear, but nurse triage, nurse prescribing, and increasing autonomy and power all help to redefine the professional role of nursing as the primary care sector develops.

Box 1.3:   Eight issues for primary care nurses

1   To consider the place for nurse leadership of primary care organisations and primary care practice.
2   To reflect on the values underpinning nursing as a profession and their continuing relevance.
3   To adapt to new roles and responsibilities – such as triage, prescribing and specialist practice while remaining true to the heritage of personal care.
4   To add value to care rather than be seen as a cheap alternative to doctor provided care.

5   To respect the place of other disciplines in the provision of care – doctors as diagnosticians, pharmacists as managers of medicines, occupational therapists and physiotherapists as specialists in supportive rehabilitation, etc.
6   To provide a fulfilling career for the new entrant as they, and the needs of the service, evolve.
7   To integrate patient care across organisational boundaries – to reduce the wall between hospital and home to a pile of rubble.
8   To redefine professionalism and professional nursing in a way that complements other caring professions.

Pharmacy

Background

The separation of pharmacists from doctors started in the eighteenth century when the growing prosperity of the population led to people buying pharmaceutical products and seeking advice about their health from chemists and drugists as well as from apothecaries.

This separation of pharmacy from the medical profession with all the associated governing arrangements, e.g. registration, control of power, accountability and supervision, developed through the pharmacy acts of the nineteenth century[19] which led to the emergence of a strong retail community pharmacy sector in the early twentieth century.

Hospital pharmacy developed with the hospital sector but had its roots in the legacy of the Poor Law hospitals and was provided either as an 'add on' to community pharmacy or as a 'stand-alone' but rather isolated service until the establishment of the NHS.

Although pharmacists' main business has traditionally been management of medicines, they have, throughout the last 200 years, also advised patients about minor ailments and undertaken tasks such as cupping and bleeding, providing surgical supplies, taking weight and blood pressure measurements, and in the past, undertaking some surgical and anaesthetic services. Thus, although the profession has separated culturally from medicine, there remain strong links between them.

The separation of the prescribing of medicines from the dispensing of them started in 1852 but became more important with the Lloyd George National Insurance Act (1911), which served to reinforce the extent to which pharmacists' incomes were dependent upon the prescribing behaviour of the medical professions.

The growth of the healthcare industry throughout the twentieth century did not leave the pharmacy profession unaffected. The social revolution following the industrial revolution, along with the tremendous growth of the multi-national pharmaceutical industry, has had profound implications. Pharmacists, as graduates, are trained in pharmacology and therapeutics and understand medicines and how they work. They are not trained to diagnose and manage medical conditions or in pathology, psychology or other aspects of medicine.

The growth of 'multiple' stores and supermarket pharmacy has led to the future of independent, retail, corner shop pharmacy being less secure. The accessibility of such pharmacies seems less attractive to the population than the economy of scale offered by supermarket pharmacies. The ending of retail price maintenance has further eroded the power base of the independent.

So the profession of pharmacy has a 200-year history of establishing itself and then adapting to the industrial and social revolutions with all their implications for the supply and management of medicines.

Clinical pharmacy in primary care

As we enter the twenty-first century pharmacists working within the primary care sector are continuing to adapt to the changing world in which they are carving out their careers. They no longer manufacture drugs, they have had much of their dispensing role automated and have remained rather isolated from the development of primary care teams and, latterly, from corporate organisations in primary care such as primary care trusts.

The development of clinical *pharmacy* services, such as those in hospitals where pharmacists are intimately involved with the provision and supervision of medicines, has been gradually developing over recent years outside hospitals in the community. Pharmaceutical advisers to health authorities and more recently primary care organisations are usually pharmacists who have had training in hospital clinical pharmacy and are aware of the potential opportunities for community pharmacists. The rapid growth in the drug budgets that the NHS faces (£6.2bn in 1999/2000) is a major driver towards the development of an effective clinical pharmacy service in the community. The implications for the profession of pharmacy are profound. No longer simply the dispenser of prescriptions and the first point of contact for advice on minor ailments, perhaps in future the pharmacist may be the manager of medicines in the primary care team, the prescriber where licensed and competent, and even the controller of the medicines budget of the primary care organisation.

Box 1.4:   Eight issues for community pharmacists

1   To end their reliance on profit from retail trade.
2   To develop as managers of medicines.
3   To support the move away from paper based prescribing systems and towards management of the supply of medicines.
4   To develop clinical pharmacy in the community.
5   To integrate clinical pharmacy practice with their hospital colleagues, so that specialist and generalist skills are available for those who need them, wherever they are.
6   To provide flexible career paths for all practitioners – to end the tyranny of being trapped by capital and the counter, the second class status of the locum and the antipathy towards PCT pharmacy advisers.
7   To reflect on the sterility of the dispensing doctor/pharmacist relationship. The profession needs to redefine its relationship with medicine, so that old battles take their rightful place in history rather than continue to get in the way of effective care.
8   To grasp the opportunities of the Crown Report[20] to develop as dependent prescribers, alongside the opportunities of local pharmaceutical schemes to expand activity into: (i) therapy support through offering medication review surgeries; (ii) drug monitoring services in diabetic and anticoagulant clinics; and (iii) and health monitoring through work with fitness centres and sports clubs.

Multiculturalism

Medicine, nursing and pharmacy represent only three of the many professional cultures involved with the provision of primary care. The heritage of the primary care sector also involves:

- dentistry
- optical services
- physiotherapy
- occupational therapy
- dietetics
- chiropody.

In addition, the close relationship between the primary care sector, other sectors of welfare provision such as social care, the voluntary sector, community and youth work and other local authority services such as environmental health and housing have played an important part in the development of the primary care sector and are likely to continue to be important for the sector's further development.

It is important to recognise that the heritage of each of these elements is different but complementary to the heritage of the whole sector (*see* Figure 1.2). Adding value to the matrix of cultures which characterise the primary care sector is the different emphasis that each puts on issues such as:

- personal and continuing care
- promoting personal autonomy
- commercial and business interests
- community interest as opposed to individual interests
- personal responsibility
- gatekeeping either to state resources or other parts of the welfare service
- democratic accountability.

While the emphases differ among all the groups involved, it is clear that the differences really matter to many of those involved and underpin many of the attitudes, values and beliefs which affect relationships and performance within the sector.

The degree of cohesion between the cultures making up the sector has to be a major interest of primary care organisations which, while reflecting on the value of what they have inherited from the past, must seek to deliver a new coherence within the sector if it is to adapt successfully to its future responsibilities.

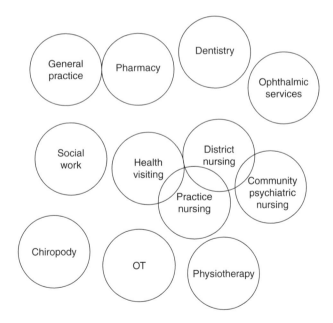

Figure 1.2:   The heterogeneous nature of the elements making up the heritage of the sector.

The task for primary care organisations of co-ordinating such provision has been likened to playing tennis with a raspberry but perhaps a better way of looking at it is illustrated in Figure 1.3.

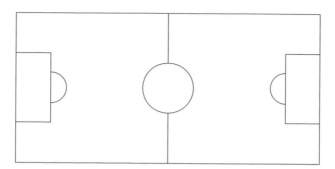

Figure 1.3:   Teamworking approach.

Rather than concentrating on the diversity of the cultural heritage, and the fact that so many of the cultures or circles relate to each other without much overlap, we must emphasise their complementary nature. All the different groups and interests involved in the primary care sector have contributed to the heritage of the sector and continue to contribute towards its success – they all play on the same 'field' – but, just as goalkeepers and centre forwards have different roles, approaches, attitudes and training programmes, so too do different players in the primary care world. The co-ordination and teamwork which distinguish an effective and successful football team from an ordinary one are just as important to success in primary care. Too often the players on the primary care field have failed to co-ordinate their efforts and been less than effective as team players.

In Figure 1.3 the idea that each of the team players can contribute their heritage to forming a successful team is illustrated. It is this teamworking approach which values each group's heritage and contribution and which primary care organisations will need to foster if the sector is to adapt successfully to its future responsibilities.

References

1 Starfield B (1994) Is primary care essential? *Lancet*. **344**: 1129–33.
2 Rivett G (1998) *From Cradle to Grave*. King's Fund, London.
3 Dawson B (1918) The future of the medical profession (Cavendish Lecture). *Lancet*. **2**: 83–5.
4 Ministry of Health Consortative Medical Council, Medical and Allied Services (1920) *Interim Report on the Future Provision of Medical and Allied Services* (Chairman Lord Dawson) CMD 693. HMSO, London.
5 Beveridge W (1942) *Beveridge Report, Parliament, Social Insurance and Allied Services*, para 428. HMSO, London.
6 Timmins N (1995) *The Five Giants*. Harper Collins, London.
7 Ministry of Health (1946) *National Health Service Bill*. Summary of the proposed new service CMD 6761. HMSO, London.
8 Ministry of Health (1948) *National Health Service Patients' Guides*. HMSO, London.

9 Collins JS (1953) Group practice. *Lancet*. **2**: 31–3; 611–15; 875–7.
10 Hadfield SJ (1953) Field survey of general practice (1951–2). *BMJ*. **2**: 683.
11 Taylor S (1954) *Good General Practice: A report on the survey*. Nuffield Provincial Hospitals Trust/Oxford University Press, London.
12 Danckwerts (1953) *Ministry of Health Report 1952*, Part 1. CMD 8933. HMSO, London.
13 Ministry of Health (1954) Future of general practice. *BMJ*. **1**: Supplement 3589.
14 Royal Commission (1966) Reports from general practice, number 5. *Evidence of the Royal Commission of Medical Education*. CGP, London.
15 Gillie A (1963) *The Field Work of the Family Doctor*. HMSO, London.
16 Illich I (1976) *Limits to Medicine, Medical Nemesis*. Penguin, London.
17 Department of Health (1997) *The New NHS: modern, dependable*. DoH White Paper, London.
18 Abel Smith B (1982) *History of the Nursing Profession*. Heinemann, London.
19 Holloway SWF (1991) *Royal Pharmaceutical Society of Great Britain 1841–1991*. The Pharmaceutical Press, London.
20 Department of Health (1999) *Review of Prescribing, Supply & Administration of Medicines*. Crown Report. DoH, London.

CHAPTER 2

The emergence of corporate primary care

Introduction

Reacting and behaving as a 'body' or corporately has not, so far, been the preferred approach of individuals and organisations making up the primary care sector. Thus far individuals and organisations in the sector have valued their autonomy and freedom to act independently – either in their own interests or on behalf of their patients/customers. Behaving corporately or 'with corporacy' implies sublimating a part of such independent autonomy to the greater good of the community and the rest of the 'corporate' organisation. In recent years the primary care sector has moved from isolated independent constituent practices and their loose association with community trusts, social service departments, pharmacies, opticians, the voluntary sector, etc. into new types of relationships. Under the umbrella of multi-funds, primary care groups, local health groups, etc., the development of corporacy within the sector has become more of a feature promoting:

- more *effective* and *efficient* provision of care – for example out-of-hours cover arrangements such as GP co-operatives, integrated nursing teams, welfare rights services in general practice and the development of intermediate care
- a more *planned* approach to service development – taking a longer term view, considering a wider range of opinions and perspectives, considering different options and piloting new ideas
- a *safer* home for a larger slice of the NHS resource – more open and accountable processes for managing finance, more support for staff committing their careers to care in the sector
- a more *accountable* service – so that the trust, so vital to effective patient care, is actively promoted rather than taken for granted.

To appreciate the challenge of developing corporacy within primary care and to understand the potential advantages and disadvantages of such behaviour it is important to appreciate how and why new, more corporate organisations are developing in the sector and how they relate to what has gone before.

This chapter explains how and why new corporate organisations are developing and the agenda they need to address if the huge cultural change is to be sustainable.[1] The alternative – the balance of power remaining with acute trusts and the new strategic health authorities (SHAs) – is a real threat if PCTs (and their equivalents outside England) fail. In this scenario the future for the values and heritage of personal, continuing, biographical, generalist and holistic care, sensitive to the needs of local communities, is bleak. Rather, a centralised, bureaucratic, performance managed, finance driven and insensitive world can be envisaged.

Power

Power within the primary care sector reflects the following.

- The ability to commit and control resources. This may be through the direct provision of care or through gatekeeping, certification, delegation or advocacy.
- Knowledge and the ability to apply that knowledge.
- Dependency through registration and behavioural norms where the professional and patient/client act in such a way as to reinforce professional power and prestige.

In the primary care sector the major consumer of resources and therefore the major seat of power is medicine and the medical profession – often referred to as the power of the 'medical model'. The sector has historically particularly focused on disease management and power within the sector reflects this focus.

GPs are in particularly powerful positions as:

- gatekeepers to specialist care, specifically trained in diagnosis and management of disease
- prescribers of effective treatments
- the profession with which the whole population registers.

Other professional groups such as nurses, dentists, pharmacists, opticians, etc. have the power of resource allocation within their areas of competence and professional knowledge. However, they do not have the power of gatekeeping (or only to a limited extent) or of a registered list (except for some dentistry) and therefore their power is inevitably more limited.

Single-handed practice

The NHS Act of 1946 provided a family doctor for everyone in the entire population, who registered with one of the 18 000 GPs making up the workforce at the time. The GPs had accepted a contract for services rendered, and remained independent practitioners, self-employed and organising their own professional lives. They were taxed as self-employed but, unlike most people in small businesses, they could not set their own fees, which were fixed and entirely dependent on the number of registrations they held, i.e. they received capitation fees. The workforce was almost entirely male, half of them were single-handed and most practised from their own homes with little or no administrative support. While the proportion of GPs who practise single-handedly has declined in response to incentives such as the group practice allowance, the ethos and culture of the autonomous GP remains. Many doctors are attracted to general practice because of the ethos of clinical freedom that exists and escape from the hierarchical management structure of the rest of the health service has been a major motivating and dynamising factor. The freedom has encompassed:

- what services to offer patients, e.g. basic general medical services or additional maternity, family planning, minor surgery, etc.
- how to offer the services, e.g. appointment systems or open access
- development of premises and employment of staff
- setting consultation hours, holiday periods, study leave and out-of-hours arrangement in consultation with local colleagues.

The freedom to develop innovative responses to local needs, to set one's own policies and standards, and stamp one's own individual personality on the practice all remain attractive. There is however a downside. Single-handed practitioners can become isolated and lack the kind of peer support and challenge which can maintain and drive up standards. While many single-handed practices have provided excellent care for many years, there has been considerable variation in standards. Lack of accountability to the community, patients and the rest of the health service for performance, behaviour and standards has been a particular problem for single-handed practice. The lack of support for single-handed practice also risks practitioner health and well-being as well as clinical standards, and the risks are increased if the practitioner dispenses medicines without pharmacy support. With a considerable number of single-handed practices having to rely on dispensing as a way of maintaining profitability, there is always the risk that practitioners may seek to maximise their profits from dispensing, rather than use the available resources on other forms of effective patient care.

Group practice

Since the 1960s more and more family doctors have grouped together as partnerships. There is no single prescribed formula or organisational structure for such partnerships and they remain as unaccountable and autonomous as single-handed general practice in their use of resources and their exercise of power. The partners are responsible for deciding on the services they will offer, providing the premises and equipment, employing staff, etc., just as single-handed practitioners are. As each partner registers patients they are each responsible for part of the income of the practice. Agreements between the partners stipulate the terms of their relationships and their responsibilities to each other and formalise arrangements between them about issues such as holidays, maternity leave, financial distribution and personal behaviour. Family doctors and practices vary greatly in the extent to which they pool their autonomy. In some cases partnerships are little more than loose alliances of single-handed practitioners who continue to behave and act with little acknowledgement of practice policies, procedures or responsibilities. In other practices the partners limit their individual freedom by agreeing a set of clinical standards and procedures, accepting individual responsibilities for areas of practice and perhaps acknowledging the special interests and expertise of partners in particular areas. Because practices have evolved in a relatively free market situation there is wide variation in the degree to which they operate in any corporate or cohesive fashion. While the role of the traditional senior partner in making all decisions, holding all financial responsibility and indeed exercising absolute power may have largely passed, nevertheless it would still be fair to say that in many cases partnership between family doctors is often not a relationship characterised by fairness, openness, accountability and mutual respect.

As the partners in the practice capitalise the practice, employ the staff, provide the premises and the equipment as well as provide the medical care, they inevitably have considerable influence over the decisions made about the development of the practice as an organisation. Meetings of partners involve decisions about allocating financial and other resources as well as decisions about service development, practice management and other issues partners may wish to raise such as the relationship between them. Inevitably, other professionals and staff working within the practice have less influence than partners over these discussions and decisions, which will tend to reflect the medical perspective of the partners in preference to other perspectives.

The primary care team

The inner team. In view of the employment and power relationships described above, it is not surprising that so many primary care teams struggle to be effective.[2] Trust and synergistic teamworking require not just acceptance of team members' professional knowledge and skill, but also respect for individuals' professional autonomy and independence. The historic dominance of medicine has seen nursing and other professions allied to medicine as less than equal and acted as a deterrent to providing maximum effective care. New members of the primary care team such as psychotherapeutic counsellors, practice nurses, etc. may have challenged the omnipotent medical mind-set but, without the power of gatekeeping and registration, have largely failed to change the team's dynamics.

The broader team. Group practices' responsibilities overlap with a large number of other workers within the primary care sector who form part of a larger primary care team. These include:

- staff traditionally employed by local authorities and community trusts such as:
  - district nurses
  - health visitors

- social services department employees such as:
  - social workers
  - community youth workers
- hospital employees such as:
  - midwives
  - dieticians
  - venisectionists
- other independent contractors such as:
  - pharmacists
  - dentists
  - opticians
- self-employed private practitioners such as:
  - physiotherapists
  - counsellors
  - osteopaths, etc.

The extent to which this broader primary care team acts in any kind of collective fashion, directed towards the common good of the community it serves, is very variable across the country but is usually very limited. Agreements across the nursing teams between practice nurses, health visitors, midwives, community psychiatric nurses, district nurses and school nurses is exceptional as they are often employed by four, if not five, separate agencies, each of which has its own priorities which its employees are expected to address. Synergistic working between the members of the extended primary care team has always been dependent upon personal relationships rather than encouraged by any incentives for effective teamworking.

This rather negative analysis should not be seen in isolation from the excellent standard of care which many primary care teams have always provided and which have marked out British family practice and primary care as one of the most developed models of effective healthcare provision in the Western world. The flexibility and dynamism of British primary care and its ability to respond to local health needs, its comprehensive population coverage and its freedom from payment at the point of provision issues, have helped it to provide high quality care despite the above constraints.

The danger of reforming the arrangements governing the working of primary care teams is that we may damage and undervalue their heritage without improving their effectiveness.

Accountability for use of resources

Since the founding of the NHS in the 1940s the primary care sector has been largely funded from general taxation but, importantly, there has been no unified allocation to support the development of *out-of-hospital services*. Rather, the development of community health services has been separated from the development of independent contractor services as a result of different funding mechanisms. Community health services have been funded through the hospital and community health service allocation (HCHS) which has also supported hospital services. All those directly employed by the health service, e.g. district nurses, received their salaries from this allocation, which also pays for the equipment, premises, hotel costs and management of NHS hospitals and community facilities. Inevitably, high profile specialist services such as the emergency, cancer and heart disease services have received greater priority than those services involved with the management of chronic disease, the elderly and mental health, and as a result the development of the community health services has been held back for many years.

Accountability for HCHS use in the community has been through the governing arrangements applying at the time. In recent years this has meant that community health services trusts have been accountable through their boards of directors to health authorities and regional offices of the NHS. Annual agreements between the trusts and health authorities replaced contracts in 1998 and form part of the service and financial framework process (SAFF) which plans and agrees investment and service development within the HCHS budget each year. Performance management through in-year monitoring of progress against the SAFF agreement involves close joint working between trusts and health authorities. Trust executive and non-executive directors are accountable for the performance and financial management of organisations and their performance is formally reported publicly through their annual reports.

Human resources form an important part of the capital of the NHS and within the community sector are particularly important as so much of the sector's work takes place in patients' homes and involves close, personal and continuing relationships with patients and their families. Employed staff, who operate under national terms and conditions of service, have access to occupational health and human resource department services operated through the employer organisations. Development of the human resource is through their employer's education and training departments, but, as has been pointed out by the Audit Commission,[3] investment in this area has not always received sufficient priority. In recent years the Non-Medical Education and Training Consortia (NMET) have commissioned both pre-registration courses and in-service training opportunities for staff spanning both the community and acute sectors. Close working relationships between providers of education such as universities, the consortia and professional bodies such as The Royal College of Nursing have helped to maintain standards. However, the lack of any systematic approach to the quality assurance of practice, as well as to education, has meant that variation in standards of care provided across the country has been large. Accountability for performance of staff has been through professional management structures, which have often reflected the priorities of the employer more than the needs of the local population or the staff member.

The independent contractor services – general practice, community pharmacy, optical services and dentistry – have been funded from general taxation through the General Medical Services (GMS) budget. This has supported the independent elements of the primary care sector and independent contractors have drawn their income from the budget once all their other expenses have been met, including items such as:

- cost of premises – capital and running costs
- staff/employment – contractors receive about 70% reimbursement of staff costs – but more staff employed means less take home pay
- management costs, such as computers, phones, electricity, etc.
- professional expenses, such as equipment, subscriptions, etc.

Inherent in this arrangement has been both the incentive for independent contractors to make the most efficient use of the resources, but also the incentive for them to maximise their income by minimising their spending.

The accountability of independent contractors for their use of resources has changed relatively little over the life of the health service. In essence, contractors have been trusted to use the resources available to them wisely. Their allocation of resources has been on an *historic use* basis and the process has been administered by a succession of authorities whose mandate has not been to performance manage or hold independent contractors accountable for their use of resources. The responsibility has been through the *executive councils (ECs), family practitioner committees (FPCs), family health service authorities (FHSAs)* and, more recently, *local health authorities (LHAs)*. Over this period of time the authorities have gradually sought to hold contractors to account for their use of financial resources more and more, in order to try to ensure quality standards, probity and equity – but their powers have always been constrained.

Independent contractors are self-employed and need to produce accounts in order to monitor their financial performance and ensure their financial health. These sets of accounts are not public documents and have never been open to scrutiny by the rest of the health service. Staff employed by independent contractors, those working with independent contractors but employed by community trusts and patients registered with independent contractors do not have access to the financial details of the contractors' performance. Some moves towards openness in this area were made through GP fundholding where the relationship between fundholding accounts and practice accounts was monitored by FHSAs and health authorities in order to ensure that funds were appropriately managed and any surpluses properly used. However, these moves were limited and ended with the end of fundholding. We have returned to the position where financial performance, profitability, policy development and implementation, organisational development and future plans are all closed books – not open to scrutiny or question, not shared with the primary care team or PCT and consequently always liable to be mistrusted.

The independent contractors also commit non-GMS resources and these are accounted for separately. Contractors commit large amounts of health service resource, prescribing budgets and resources through activities such as referral to hospital. In the year 1999/2000 the NHS spent £6.2bn on pharmaceuticals, an increase of 11.7% on the previous year and this has been increasing at between 7.3% and 14.5% every year for the last 10 years.[4] This rate of increase and size of budget have obvious implications for other budgets within the health service and indeed for the Treasury. Not surprisingly, health authorities have sought to manage their prescribing budgets more effectively through the employment of pharmacists and doctors to try to improve the clinical and cost effectiveness of prescribers' behaviour. It should be noted that this trend of increasing prescribing budgets is not restricted to the United Kingdom and indeed other countries in the Western world spend even more per patient on drugs than the United Kingdom. There has been considerable variation in prescribing costs between practitioners, practices and areas, and a great deal of work has been done by the Prescription Pricing Authority (PPA), the National Prescribing Centre (NPC) and local pharmaceutical and medical advisers to try and manage this budget more effectively. Nevertheless, the absence of any adequate incentive framework and performance management levers to change prescriber performance has made the issue problematic and this large area of public expenditure relatively undermanaged. With some GPs – dispensing doctors – relying on the supply of medicines for a large proportion of their practice profits there is an obvious perverse incentive for them to maximise their profits from supply of medicines rather than maximise their cost effectiveness.

Accountability for the use of non-financial resource in the independent contractor sector has also been less open to scrutiny than in the community sector. Human resource policies, staff development and training have been the responsibility of the independent contractor as employer and have grown in complexity as the organisations have grown and their functions expanded. While staffing and other budgets have been closely monitored by health authorities, contracts of employment, staff development and working conditions have varied considerably.

The above situation applies not only to general medical practice but also to community pharmacy, dentistry, optical services, etc. However, here the proportion of the financial and human resource that is funded by the NHS is less than in general medical practice as more is funded by co-payment from the consumer/patient. Nevertheless, the same arguments about accountability for the use of taxpayers' money apply as do the arguments about the necessity of incentive frameworks for efficiency and effectiveness and about the requirement for a performance management framework to ensure that the needs of the community and health service priorities are addressed.

In considering for example the transfer of care from hospital to home, the development of intermediate care packages, the promotion of quality in nursing and residential care, it is clear that corporate and clinical best practice are closely linked and interdependent. It should be clear that clinical power is dependent on management best practice. The inter-relationship between clinical and management power illustrated by the above is really so close that the divisions between *general management* and *clinical management* in the primary care sector and between *clinical* and *corporate governance*, while useful as an aid to thinking, may be artificial and short lived.

Responsibility

Good governance requires knowing who is responsible for what, being clear about the limits of that responsibility and ensuring that it is safe for the individual or team to hold that responsibility. Governance frameworks in the NHS emphasise the leverage for quality that governance is designed to promote, but one of the tools to deliver that quality has to be clarity about responsibility and, thus far, the frameworks have been somewhat quiet about this. It should be clear that individual patients/clients have responsibility for their own health and behaviour and at times seek to transfer that responsibility on to clinicians. Perhaps being a bit clearer about what patients and clinicians are and are not responsible for may help with their relationship! Clarity about responsibility for monitoring blood tests in patients with rheumatoid arthritis or for dealing with the results for cervical cytology screening or with questions arising about the supply chain for medicines can each illustrate the importance of responsibility. Trust in individuals and organisations is heavily dependent on being clear about who is responsible for what.

Accountability

Increasingly, individual clinicians, managers and organisations are being held to account for their performance. They are accountable to users of the service, themselves, their peers, the organisations they form part of, their professional accrediting organisation and the community. This multiplicity of accountabilities provides a framework designed to ensure that poor performance does not go unchallenged.

Contractual arrangements

The relationships between the elements of the primary care system can help to ensure good governance, quality of care and patient safety. PCTs remain accountable to the NHS and will have annual accountability agreements with the NHS Executive through *Strategic Health Authorities*. Practices, be they dental, pharmaceutical or general medical, will also have contractual arrangements with the NHS and increasingly with their local PCT, Personal Medical Services (PMS), etc. The new GP contract envisages much more local input into the contract, through which General Medical Services are provided – at least we seem to be moving towards the provision of services in primary care which better define the roles, responsibilities and powers of the parties in an open and accountable way. These agreements are important because they delineate the rules of engagement between the parties. They define who is responsible for what, the resources involved and the quality parameters. Good governance requires clarity in these issues and it will be uncomfortable for PCTs to be responsible for quality without local contracting arrangements with clinicians who are responsible for delivering that quality.

Personal development

Good governance requires that individuals who are responsible for clinical and general management are up to date and continue to provide high quality care. Ensuring access to continuing professional development, personal development and learning about best practice, should move on from being an 'anorak' pastime for enthusiasts (as it has often been in the past) to being a key corporate priority for those responsible for ensuring the primary care system operates efficiently and effectively. The introduction of *appraisal* for all clinicians is a key aspect of delivering this – through an annual, supportive and developmental approach to ensuring that all clinicians continue to develop their practice in ways which meet their own needs and those of their patients. This has already been tried in hospitals and is now being implemented for GPs and many community nurses. It needs to be extended to all clinicians, including dentists, pharmacists, therapists, counsellors and care workers if their development is to be valued and trusted.

Organisational development

The primary care sector, as much as other sectors, is made up of organisations, which need to be designed for and fit for the purpose they have to fulfil. Developing the organisations to meet their responsibilities as they change is an important part of ensuring good governance.

General practices, used to providing general medical care, will need help with organisational development to take on additional responsibilities and adapt to their changing roles:

- for health improvement
- for intermediate palliative and social care

- for specialist services such as dependency management.

Care homes, used to providing for the elderly and infirm, will also need development as organisations, if they are to provide:

- day care
- intermediate care
- rehabilitation.

To meet these new responsibilities and help their partners meet theirs, PCTs will need to develop if they are to become effective organisations and, in particular, if they are to meet their responsibilities as described in their accountability agreements with the NHS as:

- providers of care
- commissioners of care
- interpreters of the health needs of local communities
- partners in broader welfare provision.

In all areas of the primary care sector there will be similar organisational development needs that need addressing.

If these issues are to be adequately addressed then some formal organisational development programmes will be needed, in particular to meet the needs for:

- change management
- leadership
- communications
- teamworking.

Thus far, the primary care sector has been relatively excluded from NHS organisational and personal development programmes – this has to end if the sector is to safely discharge its developing new responsibilities. Otherwise the role of the sector will not be safe.[1]

Learning from experience

While much knowledge can be gained from books and study, wisdom is really only gained by tempering such knowledge with that gained from experience. Governing arrangements need to react to the real world that the organisation and clinician are experiencing and be moderated by that experience. The governance system of the organisation has to be designed to ensure that events such as 'near misses' are analysed and lessons are learnt.

Quality assurance systems

If clinicians and organisations are to be trusted by the rest of the system and by clients/patients then they need to demonstrate that they are open to scrutiny and questioning, accountable for performance and responsive to local needs and aspirations. External accreditation mechanisms such as the Royal College of General Practitioners' accreditation programmes, ISO 9000, IIP, HQS, etc. have an important function in ensuring good governance.

Through establishing the Commission for Health Improvement (CHI) the government has demonstrated its commitment to a systematic approach to quality assurance. What is required, in the primary care sector, is the necessary additional pieces of the jigsaw – quality assurance of individuals, the teams they form part of and the organisations they work for. Only then will the primary care sector be a system which the community can trust with their lives and the Treasury with its resources.

The quality assurance systems need to look at *both* clinical and corporate issues. At present most available tools look primarily at one or the other and primary care requires new tools which learn from the best elements of each.

Openness and responsiveness

If independent contractor organisations, such as GP practices, are relatively unaccountable for their use of resources and for the quality of care they provide, then, as has been discussed above, they are only one aspect of the relatively closed organisational form that independent contractor status, professional partnership, and in the case of community pharmacy, limited company status, implies. The extent to which these organisations are open to scrutiny has changed little.

- Scrutiny by health authorities has changed little. While some work openly with health authorities and welcome their input, they are often the ones whose patients stand to benefit least from such scrutiny. Practices with much to gain often resent scrutiny, fear the intrusion and questioning of their performance and face little sanction if they resist scrutiny.
- Scrutiny by patient organisations. These organisations do not have the power to enter, inspect or scrutinise the work of independent contractors and their organisations. Informal visits and liaison between community health councils (CHCs) in primary care have been encouraged, e.g. in order to develop commissioning plans under GP fundholding.[5] However, the suspicion has to remain that those who have most to gain from scrutiny and joint working with CHCs are least likely to invite participation. The extent to which patients and their representative groups can influence the policies, procedures and development plans of independent contractor organisations has never been

great. Informal suggestion schemes, patient participation groups, patient forums etc. have always been advisory and worked through informal influence rather than any power to determine resource allocation, scrutinise performance or determine policy. Patient advice and liaison services networks (PALS) may be a constructive development, but there remains the risk that they will merely be another instrument of control. They aim to guide patients on how to get the most out of a professionally controlled service rather than a channel through which patients and carers can exert more influence and some control over the services provided.

- Openness to new ideas. While many independent contractors have always been responsive to change and adaptable to new ways of working, e.g. developing the practice nurse role, practice based counselling, etc., they have been less open to new ideas that have challenged their traditional position of power. Learning lessons from clinical audit and, in particular, learning lessons from significant event audit[6] is essential if professional practice is to become safer for patients and therefore more trustworthy, but has to involve a sufficient degree of openness to external scrutiny and input to ensure that trustworthiness. The reality is that a considerable proportion of every independent contractor's work could be undertaken by others with less experience and training. While practitioners may protest about being buried in bureaucracy, drowning in patient demand and unable to take on additional work through lack of time, they may be unable to see the wood for the trees. Through opening themselves up to external scrutiny and showing a willingness to adapt to social, economic and technological change, they may have much to gain. From the public's perspective the closed nature of independent practice and its apparent antipathy to scrutiny must always raise the suspicion that it has something to fear or hide. This is damaging to the necessary trust that should exist between the caring professions and their patients/users and is damaging to the effectiveness of care.

Many practitioners will be aware that most complaints about their service relate to poor communications and management systems failures rather than clinical negligence, incompetence or irresponsibility. Unless practitioners demonstrate openly that they can learn from such complaints, change their systems and commit themselves to more open styles of communication, then the extent of the personal and organisational anguish which results from such complaints will continue. The recent review of the complaints system[7] demonstrated the extent of the required learning which practitioners and PCTs have to address.

Steps towards corporacy

Recent years have seen the gradual development of a more corporate approach to the provision of care in the sector. Fundholding encouraged general practice to develop a more collective approach to the provision of care and the commissioning of hospital services. Within each fundholding practice corporate responsibility for referral and prescribing was encouraged by the incentive of making savings which could be used for practice development. Formal review of performance by health authorities encouraged openness and joint approaches to service development, while control over some commissioning resources led to constructive consideration of care pathways between practices and local hospitals. Nevertheless, fundholding had its limitations[5] in the extent to which corporate development evolved. In addition, fundholding tended to exaggerate the differences between practices in terms of their ability to address the health needs of their communities. Non-fundholding practices often served populations with the greatest health needs but were relatively under-resourced and lacked the power of fundholders to address those health needs. Other developments within the primary care sector, such as *locality commissioning, total purchasing, out-of-hours co-operatives,* etc., can also been seen as attempts at developing a more efficient and effective sector including the development of a more corporate approach. Each of these projects and experiments relied heavily on the commitment of individuals for their success and were rarely allowed to develop over sufficient time for their lessons to be properly evaluated and their effects on the rest of welfare provision to be fully understood.

The development of primary care groups (PCGs) following the election of the Labour government in 1997[8] introduced a much more corporate approach to the primary care sector. For the first time, independent contractors and their organisations were to become part of larger, more corporate organisations. Contractors and other healthcare professionals were to have considerable power and influence over the development of these organisations but for the first time this was also to be balanced by their board including lay and social service representation alongside general and financial management expertise. PCGs and their equivalents in Scotland, Wales and Northern Ireland, have evolved rapidly in response to political pressure towards becoming autonomous PCTs. These bodies have some additional attributes of corporate organisations, such as the employment of staff, ownership of premises and provision of care as well as the commissioning of specialist services. The extent to which they succeed in fostering the development of effective primary care services through independent contractors, while at the same time encouraging corporate approaches to governance, gatekeeping and clinical quality, will be a major factor in determining their success. The extent to which independent contractors are prepared to act corporately in response to the establishment of PCTs will, undoubtedly, vary and it will be some years before we can see whether this experiment has been successful. Major investment in the primary care sector, both in terms of human resources, capital and revenue spending, has to be safe – or the Treasury, as the funder of the sector, will not trust the sector. The deal on offer would seem to be new investment for the development of more trustworthy governing arrangements including a more corporate approach to the provision and commissioning of care.

Next steps

If PCTs and their partners are to deliver on the agenda outlined in this chapter to balance the needs of patients, communities, management and clinicians, then new instruments and arrangements will need to emerge to promote delivery – and time is limited as the taxpayer's and the consumer's trust is not unlimited. Some of the instruments can be seen in the two '*futures*' outlined at www.radcliffe-oxford.com/challenge – others are being developed around the country as PCTs mature. Ideas which are emerging include the following.

- Viewing PCTs as membership organisations, which are driven by the needs of their members rather than by central dictate from the NHS Executive.
- Rationalisation of employment across practices and other PCT constituents such as integrated nursing teams, practice pharmacists, PCT employed practice nurses and counsellors, practice managers as part of a PCT management team and salaried GPs as a support for several practices facing major challenges from, for example, the homeless, drug dependent, students or immigrants.
- Tackling recruitment and retention difficulties through teaching PCT initiatives – although these, as with care trust initiatives, may need to encompass a whole health community rather than a single trust.
- Developing new contractual arrangements between the PCT and its partners – for example PMS, LPS, PDS schemes. The PCT's relationships with voluntary sector organisations and local authority departments are other examples. The questioning of existing terms of engagement can be helpful in judging issues such as the negotiations for a new GP contract[9] to replace the *Red Book* arrangements which have governed general practice for over 50 years. Box 2.1 poses the kinds of question which need to be asked of any new contract if it is to meet the needs of all the stakeholders and therefore be 'fit for purpose'. Interestingly, it could easily be argued that the same kind of approach could be taken to several other groups.

Box 2.1:   Judging any new GP contract – 10 questions

1   Does it adequately tackle the imbalance between resource need and distribution – the 'inverse care law'?
2   Does it promote and reward high quality care provision?
3   Does it challenge the 'inverse profitability' law? Does it adequately reward investment in practice development?

4   Does it ensure rapid access to professional knowledge and care when needed – and appropriately protect practitioners from inappropriate demand?

5   Does it promote a more open and accountable relationship between practitioners and patients, staff and primary care team members so that they all feel important and valued members of the organisation?

6   Does it promote a coherent approach between practice policies and the PCT's policies? Does it support a robust and supportive relationship between them?

7   Does it develop an appropriately flexible career package for GPs – as their desire for varying degrees of commitment, development of special interests, moving between practices, investing capital and taking time out requires?

8   Does it tackle poor performance in a way which maintains the trust of all parties, values knowledge and experience but challenges arrogance, lack of skills or knowledge, professional isolation and demotivation?

9   Does it break down the rigid barriers to the provision of care across organisational boundaries – encourage GPs to care for their patients in hospital as well as work with specialist colleagues as they care for patients at home – to avoid emergency admissions where appropriate and to shorten waiting times and lists by providing more care themselves?[10]

10   Does it make it safe for taxpayers to trust practitioners, not just with their lives, but also with their money? Does it encourage sound governance, confidential care, open books, accountable performance and sensitive use of clinical power?

References

1 Department of Health (2002) *Shifting the Balance of Power: the next steps.* DoH, London.
2 West M and Slater J (1996) *Teamworking in Primary Health Care. A review of its effectiveness.* HEA, London.
3 Audit Commission (2001) *Hidden Talents.* Audit Commission, London.
4 *Script* (2001) **2621:** 5.
5 Audit Commission (1996) *What the Doctor Ordered.* Audit Commission, London.
6 Department of Health (2000) *An Organisation with a Memory.* DoH, London.
7 York Health Economics Consortium (2001) *NHS Complaints Procedure National Evaluation.* YHEC, York.
8 Department of Health (1997) *The New NHS: modern, dependable.* DoH White Paper, London.
9 GMC/NHS Confederation (2002) *The New GMS Contract.* GMC, London.
10 NHS Alliance (2002) *Vision in Practice.* NHS Alliance, London.

CHAPTER 3

The governance of primary care

Introduction

As the primary care sector has evolved and developed over the first 50 years of the NHS in the United Kingdom, so the patchwork of arrangements through which the sector is governed has changed. In the past the sector was administered, managed, directed and governed so as to ensure both the safety of patients receiving care within the sector and the safety of funds spent within the sector or committed through the sector. This is no longer a sufficiently robust set of arrangements and this chapter explores why and what response is needed. The arrangements need to reflect the interests of all the stakeholders in the sector but historically have not necessarily balanced their interests in ways which adequately reflect the developing responsibilities of the sector.

While considerable recent attention has been devoted to describing and developing the arrangements through which clinical care can be 'quality assured' in a framework of clinical governance, similar consideration and development are also required of the organisational and corporate processes which underpin safe governance in the sector.

Although for the sake of clarity, clinical and corporate governance will be described and discussed separately, it should be appreciated that they are in reality different aspects of the same system and that they are *interdependent*.

Corporate governance

In introducing their 'code of best practice', the Cadbury Committee[1] described the principles on which that code was based. These principles are those of openness, integrity and accountability.

Openness on the part of companies – with which the Cadbury Report is concerned – is within the limits set by their competitive position. It is the basis for the confidence that needs to exist between the business and all those who have a stake in its success. An open approach to the disclosure of information contributes to the efficient working of the market economy, prompts boards to take effective action and allows shareholders and others to scrutinise companies more thoroughly. Through these considerations openness promotes confidence in the company by reducing any suspicion that the company has anything to hide.

Integrity means both straightforward dealing and completeness. What is required of financial reporting is that it should be honest and present a balanced picture of the state of the company's affairs. The integrity of reports depends on the integrity of those who prepare and present them.

Boards of directors are **accountable** to their shareholders and both have to play their part in making that accountability effective. Boards of directors need to do so through the quality of information provided to shareholders and shareholders through their willingness to discharge their responsibilities as owners. Non-executive directors act as representatives of the shareholders on the board and have the responsibility to hold the executive to account at board meetings. Corporate scandals, such as the Poulson affair and in more recent times the Emron crash, have served to focus attention on this key role for non-executive directors.

Interpreting these principles through a code of best practice has been important in maintaining the essential trust that is required between limited companies, their shareholders and their customers.

The extent to which the same principles and code can be transferred to the primary care sector within the NHS needs consideration. The taxpayer and the patient are analogous to the shareholder and the customer of limited companies while the patchwork of independent contractors, community services, local authority services, voluntary sector agencies and private sector providers is analogous to the companies that the code of best practice refers to.

In introducing the principles on which the code of best practice is based, the Cadbury Committee considered two main arguments.

1   A clear understanding of the responsibilities involved in governing the companies and an open approach to the way in which these responsibilities have been discharged would assist the directors in framing and winning *support* for their strategies.
2   Clarity would assist the efficient operation of business and the level of confidence in boards, auditors and financial reporting and hence the general level of *confidence* in business.

Box 3.1:   Case study – A partnership with problems

Mohamed, David and Jane had been the partners at Grove Street for over 15 years; they owned the surgery, employed the staff, dispensed the drugs and worked hard. They have never really agreed about things – David wanted to provide quality care, while Jane was more interested in an easy life and Mohamed put most of his energy into his clinical assistant post in dermatology. Their list has been falling – another local practice seems to be more popular and a complaint about Jane's handling of a local problem family received wide adverse publicity. A relationship between one of the receptionists and a local pharmacist and a row between David and the local GP co-operative executive have not helped to enhance working relationships.

The confidence of the partners in each other, of patients and staff in the practice and of the PCT in the potential of the practice has been damaged by the partners' failure to direct the business, to understand their responsibilities and the importance of good relationships. The closed nature of the partnership model and their failure to communicate, support each other and develop the business have not helped.

The result – yet another dysfunctional practice failing to provide the kind of healthcare their knowledge, skills and resources should permit. A practice failing its patients, failing its partners and its staff.

The arguments for adhering to similar principles and to a similar code of practice in the primary care sector are essentially the same.

1   A clearer understanding of their responsibilities by the parties involved in governing the primary care sector (the taxpayer as funder, the patient or customer as consumer and the organisations, both directors and staff) and of the relationship between all of them, will help to re-establish the *confidence* of all parties in the system.

2   A more open approach to the relationship between the parties along with a more open approach to the sharing of financial and management information will help build confidence between the parties and ensure *support* for developments.

The Cadbury Committee also considered that if standards of financial reporting and business conduct were not seen to be raised, a greater reliance on regulation would be inevitable. They also considered that any further degree of regulation would, in any event, be more likely to be well directed, if it were to enforce what has already been shown to be workable and effective by those setting the standards. In the primary care sector, the extension of regulation through both individual professional re-accreditation and processes of organisational quality assurance is more likely to be well directed if it reinforces accepted best practice in both individual and organisational processes.

The extent to which organisations within the primary care sector meet the standards in the Cadbury Report's code of best practice ought to be considered – but in the context of a clinical, professional and care oriented environment as compared to a commercial one.

•   We have to appreciate that the extent to which each of the standards is relevant in the primary care sector does vary with circumstances and that they have to reflect both the confidential nature of the relationships involved in clinical practice and the very different relationship characteristics which exist when we are healthy compared to when we are sick.

- The confidence and trust the parties need to have in clinical practice and the necessary dynamic relationship between clinical and management power that is required for effective clinical practice is an extension of the confidence and trust considered by Cadbury.
- That integrity is at least as important to confidence in clinical practice as it is in commercial practice.

We will consider each element in turn.

The board of directors

The Board shall meet regularly, retain a full and effective control over the company and monitor the executive management.

*Cadbury**

Within the primary care sector, there have been a variety of boards of directors who have determined the pattern of services available within the sector in any locality. Until the development of PCGs and PCTs (and analogous primary care organisations in Scotland, Wales and Northern Ireland), there has been no corporate approach to providing direction to the primary care sectors and no one board to retain full or effective control. Boards of directors, be they GPs or other independent contractors, directing their own organisations, voluntary sector or local authority sector bodies, community trusts or private sector providers, such as the owners of nursing and residential care homes, have all had separate governing arrangements. Each of them will have had managing boards which have met regularly and which have retained full and effective control over their individual organisations, and monitored the discharge of their responsibilities through their executive arm. What has not happened until recently has been any effective co-ordination of their provision and, indeed, even at the present time, the extent to which PCGs, PCTs, etc. can direct and determine provision within their area is limited. This patchwork of arrangements for the provision of care provides great local sensitivity to differing needs, but may perpetuate historic unfairness in provision and variation in the extent to which boards retain full and effective control over provision.

There should be clearly accepted division of responsibilities at the head of the company, which will ensure a balance of power and authority, such that no one individual has unfettered powers of decision. Where the Chairman is also the Chief Executive, it is essential that there should be a strong and independent element on the board, with a recognised senior member.

---

*Subsequent displayed quotations between pp 42 and 46 are from the Cadbury Report.

In the primary care sector, there has clearly been a separation and division of responsibilities between the independent contractor organisations so that there is now no possibility of excessive power being held within one individual or board. There have, however, been individuals with unfettered powers of decision within constituent organisations in the sector, where independent contractors such as GPs have been the executive directors of their organisations, the main face-to-face providers of care, and the owners and capitalisers of the business. There has really been no clearly accepted division of responsibilities within the organisations, as necessary to ensure a balance between power and authority. This has placed the individual independent contractor in a privileged, but exposed position.

> The board should include non-executive directors of sufficient calibre and number for their views to carry significant weight over the board's decision.

Within the primary care sector, there has, until recently, been no role for non-executive directors except in private sector limited companies. The appointment of lay members to PCGs and non-executive directors to PCT boards has introduced this element into the sector, so that the views of the community and shareholders (the taxpayers) are given significant weight, sufficient to enable them to challenge the executive's power.

> The board should have a formal schedule of matters specifically reserved to it for decision to ensure that the direction and control of the company is firmly in its hands.

Once again, this degree of formality in board processes has not been a characteristic of the primary care sector thus far. While independent contractors' organisations will have operated within partnership agreements and local arrangements for decision making, these have not been systematically arranged and have not dealt in any formal way with determining who needs to decide what in which particular circumstances. There is then always the risk that integrity will be jeopardised and accountability be too loose.

> There should be an agreed procedure for directors in the furtherance of their duties to take independent professional advice if necessary at the company's expense.

This necessary check on the power of the executive, whereby directors can seek independent advice, has not been a characteristic of the design of the governing arrangements in primary care. While agreements between independent contractors in an organisation may well describe the circumstances where independent financial and legal advice could be sought, this has not been seen as any kind of check or balance mechanism on the executive.

> All directors should have access to the advice and services of the company secretary, who is responsible to the board for ensuring the board procedures are

followed and that applicable rules and regulations are complied with. Any question of the removal of the company secretary should be a matter for the board as a whole.

Arrangements vary in the different organisations within the primary care sector. Within local authorities and community trusts, the arrangements have often been analogous. Within the voluntary sector and independent contractual organisations, the necessary company secretary functions have largely been fulfilled by voluntary sector officers and practice managers. The extent to which boards have delegated powers to them and held them accountable for the discharge of their responsibilities has varied greatly. Practice managers have often fulfilled this role in general practice, but their position has always been vulnerable to the power of partners acting individually or as a group.

Non-executive directors

Non-executive directors should bring an independent judgement on the issues of strategy, performance, resources including key appointments and standards of conduct.

In the absence of non-executive directors, there has been little independent judgement on these matters within the sector but the advice of health authorities, patients and independent advisers has frequently been sought over such key issues – although key appointments, such as GPs, are seldom subject to this kind of external independent judgement. It will take some time for non-executive directors of PCTs to have sufficient confidence in each other for their independent role to be valued.

The majority should be independent of management and free of any business or other relationships, which could materially interfere with the exercise, apart from their fees and shareholding. Their fees should reflect the time which they commit to the company.

In the absence of non-executive directors, this may seem to be irrelevant in the primary care sector but, nevertheless, this necessary check on the exercise of power by the executive board has been important. The necessary check has largely been through the exposure of the executive to patient influence and through the monitoring of performance by health authorities and trusts who are free of the kind of financial bias involved.

Non-executive directors should be appointed for specific terms and reappointment should not be automatic.

This has applied to lay members and PCGs and non-executive directors of the PCTs and limited companies within the sector as well as the non-executive members of health authorities and community trusts.

Non-executive directors should be selected through a formal process and both this process and their appointment should be a matter for the board as a whole.

Again, this applies as above.

Executive directors

Directors' service contracts should not exceed three years without stakeholders' approval.

Independent contractors are not constrained by short-term contracts and it has always been considered that the requirement for continuity of care and commitment to building up long-term relationships with patients has been of overriding importance. The power of independent contractors resulting from their registered list, knowledge base and ownership of the business has always been seen to outweigh the advantages of increased accountability that short service contracts would introduce. In these terms, the greater power consequent upon long-term appointments has to be balanced by greater accountability and openness.

There should be full and clear disclosure of directors' total emoluments and those of the chairman and highest paid UK director, including pension contributions and stock options. Separate figures should be given for salary and performance related elements and the basis on which performance is measured should be explained.

This has applied to community trusts and health authorities as well as limited companies within the sector and will apply to primary care trusts. Among independent contractor organisations, this degree of openness has never been required. The lack of such a requirement and the lack of openness does, of course, fail to damp down speculation about the variation in emoluments that exists. This lack of openness is increasingly out of line with best practice elsewhere and is damaging to the image of the professions concerned.

Executive directors' pay should be subject to the recommendations and remuneration committee made up of wholly or mainly executive directors.

Again, this is applied in health service and local authority bodies but not among independent contractors.

Reporting and controls

It is the board's duty to present a balanced and understandable assessment of the company's position.

There has been no requirement for any independent contractor organisation to present a balanced and understandable assessment of their organisation's position to either customers, i.e. patients, or shareholders such as health authorities. Reports regarding performance, such as referral and prescribing, have been required as part of GP fundholding or PMS contracts, but these are exceptional and never present a full, balanced and understandable assessment of the performance of the contractor and organisation. They have always been limited to specific parts of the organisational performance and have never dealt with all aspects of the organisation's financial performance.

> The board should ensure that an objective and professional relationship is maintained with the auditors.

Independent contractor businesses will have a professional relationship with their accountants but these fall short of those required for limited companies in that the contractor's accounts do not have to be formally audited.

> The board should establish an audit committee of at least 3 non-executive directors with terms of reference which deal clearly with its authority and duties.

This is not a requirement in the primary care sector among independent contractors, although it is complied with by health authorities and community trusts as well as local authorities.

> The directors should explain the responsibility for preparing the accounts next to a statement by the auditors about their reporting responsibilities.

Again, this is not a requirement for independent contractors or the voluntary sector.

> The directors should report on the effectiveness of the company's systems of internal controls.

Controls assurance is being introduced into primary care along with the rest of the health service but has not characterised arrangements up until now.

> The directors should report that the business is a going concern with supporting assumptions or qualifications as necessary.

Again, this follows from the introduction of controls assurance and an open reporting style which has not, thus far, been characteristic of the sector.

It can be seen from the above that the extent to which primary care provider organisations, such as independent contractor partnerships, have enjoyed a privileged position is very considerable, and that for the most part this position has been justified by the quality of service and care that has been provided.

However, it is now apparent that the customer and shareholder, i.e. the patient and the taxpayer, no longer retain a sufficient degree of trust in the quality of that performance, to continue with *all* elements of this privileged position. A greater degree of *openness, accountability and responsiveness* is now required of all elements within the primary care sector, if they and the sector are to continue to be trusted with the power that the sector has previously enjoyed. The introduction of the necessary checks and balances to make the discharge of this power safe is now being demanded of the sector through proposals for peer review, quality assurance, accountability and openness.

While we have mainly considered the financial aspects of corporate governance as elegantly described in the Cadbury Report,[1] these can only be one part of the corporate governance framework, which the primary care sector needs to espouse for the future. Corporate governance, or the arrangements governing corporate behaviour within the sector, is essentially a consideration of the safe and effective discharge of corporate power. Figure 3.1 illustrates the relationships involved.

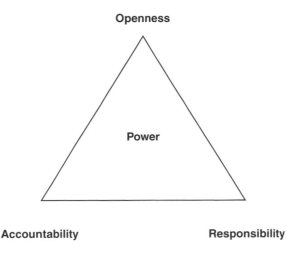

Figure 3.1:   Relationships in corporate governance.

Openness

In addition to openness about financial issues and performance, decision-makers in the primary care sector will also need to consider openness in other areas.

- Their policy decision-making processes regarding the provision of primary care services and their commissioning of specialist secondary care services.
- Being open about their decisions, why they have made them and how they have been influenced to make those decisions is an important aspect of building trust in the decision-making process. If making better decisions requires better processes for making the decisions, then openness in the decision-making process is an important element.

It is not just in making better decisions that good governance in primary care requires a greater degree of openness. Openness is also required in relationships both within organisations in the sector, and between the organisations making up the sector. Too often, organisations within the sector have deaf ears to the voices of staff, patients, customers, health services management, etc. concerning their behaviour and, as a result, the confidence that all parties have in elements of the sector has been harmed.

Box 3.2

The local PCG, along with many others, had sought the views of a random sample of patients about their experience of the care provided by their practice (using the GPAS survey tool).[2] The results were both numerical and descriptive, and were reported back to the practices as a way of helping them decide how to improve their service. The issue of whether to share the numerical information between practices, so they could compare their performance with similar local practices, exercised the PCG board for some time. Eventually all practices were consulted and as a result the board agreed to 'break the code' and let all the practices have all the numerical data. The issue revolved around the added value and increased opportunity for learning and development that openness and sharing offered. Increasingly the 'closed' approach is changing: prescribing data, referral data, patient satisfaction data – where next? Possibly other aspects of clinical performance and then financial performance.

Accountability

Being held to account for decisions made, behaviour, use of resources and development is another important element in maintaining the trust between organisations in the primary care sector and between that sector and its customers and shareholders. While being open also implies being open to suggestion, open to criticism and open to new ideas, being accountable also implies:

- justifying performance both in making decisions and in implementing the consequences of those decisions
- demonstrating how individuals and organisations have changed as a result of being held to account for their performance
- answering questions about performance both during the process of decision making and during the implementation of those decisions. With most decisions in primary care being made by the executive boards without the involvement of non-executive directors, this process of accountability is weakened. Accountability during the decision-making process is reduced by not having non-executive involvement and also by executive decisions not being open to challenge by other stakeholders such as health authorities, PCTs, etc. – when this element of accountability is lacking, then trust in both the implementation and in the organisation is threatened.

Responsiveness

The extent to which individuals, organisations and the primary care sector are responsive to both national policy and local individual need and can illustrate how that responsiveness is an important element in demonstrating sound governance. Failure to respond to either national policy issues such as health and safety or human resource best practice, or local needs such as premises improvement, staff development or patient complaints regarding attitudes or accessibility is deeply damaging. Lack of responsiveness reduces the confidence that stakeholders have in the governing arrangements of the sector. Even if most individuals and organisations are responsive most of the time, it is like a rotten apple in a barrel – poor practice affects everyone's reputation.

Power

Each of the above elements has to be satisfactorily addressed if all stakeholders are to have confidence that power within the primary care sector is being safely and effectively discharged. Power in the sector comes from a number of sources.

- *From knowledge.* In the case of corporate power in the primary care sector, this knowledge relates to the history, dynamics, relationships and potential within the sector.
- *Control over resource allocation.* In the past, the majority of resources within the health service flowed between health authorities and secondary care trusts, those within primary care were junior partners in this relationship. The introduction of PCTs and the changes to the design of the primary care sector[3] have meant that primary care will be responsible for committing over 75% of health service resources. This change is illustrated in Figure 3.2 and with the associated changes at health authority level it is likely that even more than 75% will be under the control of primary care organisations. When the power of resource allocation involves not only the commissioning of hospital care but also the provision of primary care services, then perhaps independent contractors, whose income is dependent on profits from the provision of primary care, should declare an interest in how those resources are spent.

Up until now, independent contractor organisations within primary care have had the trust of the public in how they use the resources at their disposal but with the increase in resource allocation power must come an increase in openness, accountability and responsiveness if that trust is to be maintained.

Relationships

Sound governance in the primary care sector is as dependent on relationships within the sector and between the sector and the rest of welfare services, as is

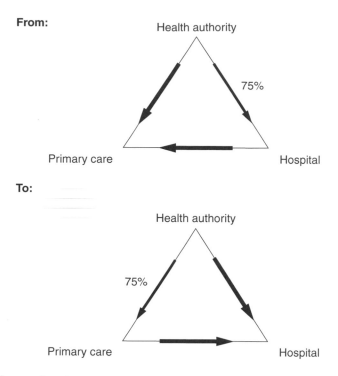

Figure 3.2:   Changes in primary care.

governance in any other sector. In considering the governance of nations in the *Book of Common Prayer* or between nations in the establishment of the United Nations or the development of the European Union, the relationships between constituents are always central to effective governance. Considering the development of the European Union can help to illuminate some of the issues relevant to the primary care sector.

Europe has developed as a group of separate nation states which have not always agreed with each other about important issues and this has led in the past to world wars and unmeasurable suffering. The coming together of these nation states into the European Union has required them to re-examine their relationships and how and in what circumstances they share power between them. The recent white paper on European governance[4,5] examines these governance issues with particular emphasis on the expansion of the Union and the power of the Commission Parliament and nation states. The analogy to the expanding power of the primary care sector and the powers of the individual practitioner, practice and PCT, is worthy of consideration.

Closer co-operation between nation states might, for example, help member states try to cope with the problems of reforming pension funding so as to develop common solutions, even if these would not apply to other member states which rely on state financed basic pensions or self-funded public or private pensions.

Similarly, co-operation between member states with national health systems might help them find common solutions to increasing demand and demographic forces, which would not apply in countries relying on private finance or insurance funded systems. Closer co-operation and the exploration of potential common solutions is an instrument for the development of the European Union, which allows considerable power to remain with the nation state, and is thus not particularly attractive to a 'centralist commission' approach.

Open co-ordination goes much further in accommodating diversity in the approach of nation states but holds such diversity within a relationship between that nation state and the Commission where the freedom of action and the areas for independent action are agreed and where the lessons learnt from performance are freely shared and learnt by all nation states.

The relationship between independent contractor organisations and between them and corporate primary care organisations, such as PCTs, is analogous. Until recently, the organisations had great autonomy as did nation states, but in the new world where lessons have been learnt from the past and the sector has increased in power, then these relationships need to be reconsidered. Closer co-operation between practitioners can be an instrument for improving performance where there are particular common issues that they face, such as prescribing overspends or staff training. Open co-ordination between the PCT and its constituent organisations could help to ensure that the development and implementation of best practice is efficiently and effectively co-ordinated.

What would seem to be required for the development of good governance within the primary care sector is a fundamental re-think of the roles, responsibilities and relationships involved within the sector. The safe exercise of power by the sector and the trustworthiness of the sector depend on finding answers to the questions raised which satisfy all the parties and promote trust between them.

Clinical governance

A new system in NHS Trusts and primary care to ensure that clinical standards are met, and that processes are in place to ensure continuous improvement, backed by new statutory duty for quality in NHS Trusts.[4]

- Clinical governance is a new system for improving the standard of clinical practice. It is a new framework to improve the quality of care incrementally over the years. This framework challenges clinicians' traditional individual autonomy and sees them as part of a system; it will only succeed to the extent that clinicians find it supportive and helpful.
- Existing activities, such as clinical audit, education and training, research and development and risk management (including complaints) will each become part of the clinical governance framework. The approach will be

systemic, with a senior clinician responsible for clinical governance through-out each organisation, and an important link to planning processes such as the health improvement programmes, accountability agreement and personal organisational development planning.

- The chief executive of an NHS trust or health authority, as the accountable officer, will have responsibility for quality including clinical governance.
- The system will be open to public scrutiny – it will be reported on at board meetings and subject to an annual reporting cycle.
- The system is not fixed and will need to evolve over time to take into account changes in the accreditation processes, development and partnership working, and changes to funding streams such as those brought about by the development of workforce confederations.

While earlier in this chapter corporate governance was considered as the system through which the corporate behaviour of organisations is governed, so clinical governance should now be considered in an analogous way as the system through which the clinical behaviour and performance of individual clinicians and the organisations they form part of are governed. While much attention has been focused on the clinical performance of individual clinicians and the governing arrangements of it, we also need to consider the arrangements governing team and organisational clinical performance. As with corporate governance, these are the arrangements which *make it safe* for patients to put their trust and their lives in the hands of clinicians' teams and organisations, safe for the clinicians to devote their working lives to the organisations and safe for the community to trust the individuals and organisations with the responsibility of treating disease and maintaining health.

The elements of clinical governance can be illustrated as in Figure 3.3.

Education

In the modern health service, it is no longer acceptable for any clinician to abstain from continuing education after qualification – too much of what is learned during training becomes outdated too quickly. Different systems have emerged to support continuing professional development by different practitioner groups – for example, post registration education and practice (PREP) for nurses, post graduate education allowance (PGEA) for GPs, continuing professional development (CPD) for hospital and community trusts' doctors. Some practitioners have become trained educators to support such approaches (for example, GP tutors and clinical practice nurse tutors). In addition, some specialities such as medical specialities and specialist nursing have a requirement for considerable periods of post-graduate study before accreditation. For other practitioner groups, such as pharmacists, physiotherapists and occupational therapists, education has been a responsibility of the employer and the relevant professional body.

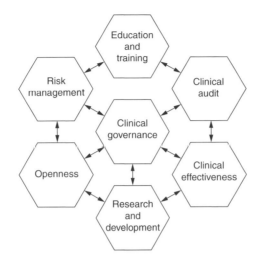

Figure 3.3:   The elements of clinical governance.

Most of this educational activity has been focused on the individual practitioner and his or her own practice; the need to educate groups of practitioners together for the roles they fulfil together has not been well addressed. One of the reasons has been the way education has been funded. Medical and dental education, undergraduate, postgraduate and continuing professional development have been funded through the medical and dental education levy (MADEL) funding stream, while non-medical education has been funded through the NMET funding stream. These two funding streams have dealt with clinical education and development, but the needs of other staff such as managers and administrative staff and indeed all those directly employed by independent contractors, such as practice nurses, have been less secure. These administrative staff and practice-employed staff have depended on their employers to fund education and this has often been supported by health authority local arrangements. The cost of releasing employed staff, such as practice nurses, has often fallen on independent contractors who are faced with the difficult dilemma of investing in their staff education at the expense of their profits.

The recent development of NHS workforce confederations brings together the different funding streams to support the education and development of the whole primary care workforce. The formation of the *University of the National Health Service* is also designed to boost in-service training and respond to the criticisms of workforce education and development, highlighted in the recent reports of the Audit Commission.[6] The success of these confederations in addressing the educational and development needs of individuals – clinicians and non-clinicians working in the primary care sector – will depend on their ability to balance the interests of individuals and the organisations of which they are part. In addition, the confederations will need to manage change in the balance of education and training away from processes which support separate development of individuals and professions and towards those which support team and organisational development as they have received less attention in the past. The extent and speed at which educational providers are able to adapt and respond to the evolving needs of the primary care sector will also need to be managed by the confederations. In a world of rapid technological change, the opportunities and challenges for workforce development demand both an informed questioning of current provision and a more dynamic approach to planning future provision.

We can anticipate PCTs providing education and training programmes for staff or commissioning them jointly with other PCTs using funds from their unified budgets and also wanting to develop a relationship with workforce confederations so that they commission programmes of relevance to the identified and agreed needs of the PCT. The extent to which they have control or influence over the activities of the confederations is unclear at present, but as the major controlling party of NHS resources, it would seem inevitable that they will become, at least, influential in this area.

As illustrated in Figure 3.3, education and training have to be informed by, and inform, the other elements of clinical governance so that the provision is informed by issues arising from clinical audit, complaints, new evidence on clinical effectiveness or from R&D programmes and similarly informs their evolution. So the outcome of education programmes – the new learning resource – can change organisational as well as individual attitudes and performance.

Box 3.3:   Education and training in service development

In the local health authority area, an audit of the cervical cytology screening programme showed a particularly high level of 'inadequate smears'. More detailed audit identified issues for those who take smears as well as those who organise their transport and analysis. A systematic approach to providing additional education and training for all those parties involved in the programme was implemented as a result of the audit and is leading to considerable improvement in performance. As a result of the education programme, practitioners who take relatively few smears, such as some general practitioners, are being encouraged by those who have been on the retraining programme to stop taking smears or retrain.

This approach to seeing education and training as part of service development and quality assurance, i.e. as a clinical governance lever, has many positive benefits, not least to those women whose anxiety and worry about the results of their smear tests is only heightened by having to be frequently recalled, simply because of an inadequate smear result.

Clinical audit

Clinical audit is the review of clinical performance, the refining of clinical practice as a result and the measurement of performance against agreed standards – a cyclical process of improving the quality of clinical care. In one form or another, audit has been part of good clinical practice for generations. Participation in audit has been a requirement of NHS trust employees, including doctors, and protected time has been provided. However, participation has only been *encouraged* in primary care where audit time has had to compete with other priorities and has not been directly funded or had identified time given to it.

Audit has been facilitated by trained staff and committees in NHS trusts and through groups such as the medical audit advisory groups (MAAGs) in primary care. Although initially regarded as a medical prerogative, in recent years audit activity has spread to include other members of the clinical team as well as patients and managers where appropriate. Many audit protocols are available 'off the shelf' for commonly performed projects and the data collection and analysis requirements are handled by the administrative staff. Funding for clinical audit has varied from place to place, depending on the priority health authorities and NHS trusts have given it. Management cost pressures have made it difficult to sustain a comprehensive programme of clinical audit activity, particularly in primary care where audit has not been underpinned by contractual arrangements.

Medical audit has moved to become clinical audit just as other practitioner groups' perspectives have been noted as essential to quality improvement. In primary care, clinical audit has also frequently involved the users' perspective and health authorities have supported this process and encouraged NHS trusts to adopt a similar approach.

Participation in clinical audit has increasingly been used as a lever in attempts by funders to improve clinical quality. Access to funds for service development has been dependent on clinical audit activity through schemes such as GP fundholding, PMS and prescribing incentive schemes. However, the extent to which such activity has been part of a systematic approach to improving the quality of care patients receive has been limited. Rather, participation has been accepted as sufficient evidence and in future we will need to look more at the lessons learnt and change rather than simply participation will need to be implemented.

As illustrated in Figure 3.3, clinical audit needs to have a dynamic relationship with the other elements of clinical governance.

Clinical effectiveness

Clinical effectiveness is a measure of the extent to which a particular intervention works. The measure on its own is useful, but it is enhanced by considering whether the intervention is appropriate and whether it represents value for money. In the modern health service, clinical practice needs to be refined in the light of emerging evidence of effectiveness but also has to consider aspects of efficiency and safety from the perspective of the individual patient and carers in the wider community.

Clinical effectiveness also struggles to measure some of the qualitative aspects of care that a broader definition of care needs to encompass. These include issues such as continuity of care, care which is sensitive to the personal needs of the patient and care which is based on an holistic analysis of the individual patient's needs, rather than the effectiveness of any particular intervention.

Clinical effectiveness has been promoted through the development of guidelines and protocols for particular diseases. These are based on evidence of effectiveness as assessed following randomised controlled trials, meta-analyses and systematic reviews, and made more understandable by the use of terminology such as 'numbers needed to treat' (NNTs).

The natural conservativism of clinical practitioners inevitably leads to a delay in the implementation of new evidence of effective practice. Clinical guidelines, protocols, etc., along with publications such as *Effectiveness Bulletins* and *Bandolier*, have been attempts to encourage adoption of the evidence of effective care and this has been further developed through formal guidance from the National Institute for Clinical Excellence (NICE), which has attempted to weigh the evidence of clinical and cost effectiveness and produce guidance for the NHS.

Unfortunately, such guidance is always open to criticism by those who feel threatened, either because the guidance implies their need to change, to spend or to save money. In addition, we have to realise that clinical and cost effectiveness measures are never absolute and may sometimes conflict. The needs of individual patients are not the same as the needs of populations and the task of the clinician is never simply to weigh up the balance between these elements. Those responsible for clinical governance are likely to encourage the development of clinical practice in the light of clear evidence of effectiveness and to encourage the adoption of guidance, such as NICE recommendations. The extent to which such guidance is used as leverage for changing clinical practice and the effectiveness of such leverage is yet to be determined. The medico-legal implications of the adoption of effective practice or failure to adopt it should not be forgotten. Practitioners are increasingly being asked to justify their clinical practice and the clinical governance framework is likely to make this process of justification more open and explicit. Practitioners who do not follow recommendations will need to be able to justify their position and document their reasons. As Figure 3.3 illustrates, the relationship between clinical effectiveness and the other elements of clinical governance is important. Evidence of clinical effectiveness on its own does not improve the quality of care patients receive. It can only be through education, audit, risk management, etc. that the evidence of effectiveness can change behaviour and improve the quality of care.

Risk management

Providing healthcare is a risky business. There are risks to the patient, risks to the practitioner and risks to the provider organisation. These risks all need to be minimised as part of any quality assurance programme.

- *Risk to patients*. Compliance with statutory regulations can help to minimise risks to patients. Examples are the Data Protection Act, the Control of Substances Hazardous to Health (COSHH) Regulations, Medicines Control Agency approval, indemnity insurance and so on. In addition, patient risks can be minimised by ensuring that systems are regularly reviewed and questioned – for example, by critical event audit and learning from complaints.
- *Risks to practitioners*. Ensuring that clinicians are immunised against infectious diseases, work in a safe environment and are helped to keep up to date are important parts of quality assurance. In the past, the levers to ensure good practice have been stronger in the NHS trusts than in primary care, and it is anticipated that the clinical governance framework will encourage wider dissemination of good practice.
- *Risks to the organisation*. Poor quality is a threat to any organisation. In addition to reducing risks to patients and practitioners, organisations need to reduce their own risks by ensuring high quality employment practice (including locum procedures and reviews of individual and team performance), a safe environment (including estates and privacy) and well designed policies on public involvement.

Associated organisations such as GP co-operatives, community pharmacists and residential care homes, should be covered by the clinical governance framework by agreeing to comply with the standards of the organisations with which they are associated.

Box 3.4:   Case study – Care of the elderly

Mildred is 90, resident in a local private nursing home, physically frail and a bit forgetful.

She suffers from diabetes, cardiac failure, hypothyroidism and takes a regular cocktail of 12 different drugs.

She is cared for by the nursing staff, visited by her general practitioner whenever a crisis arises and is also visited by a local pharmacist who keeps an eye on her medication. She still visits her optician and chiropodist as well as hospital outpatients about her diabetes, heart failure and anticoagulant therapy.

Joe joins the local practice as a GP registrar and as part of his training carries out an audit of diabetic care in the elderly. He meets Mildred and decides to look at the quality of healthcare she is receiving. Although every one of the 18 clinicians involved is well motivated, competent and caring, they:

- don't know each other

- have never talked to each other about Mildred's care
- are employed by 10 different organisations, each with its own set of clinical policies and priorities
- have never studied or learnt together
- are only aware of best practice within their own specialism or profession.

Joe talks to the local clinical governance group at the PCT. Mildred's care raises many issues, but for the group it is the difficulty of ensuring best clinical practice and care across professional, organisational, private sector/NHS boundaries which poses the most difficult questions. If clinical governance means anything for Joe and Mildred it has to address the quality of care received by the most vulnerable and most needy. For Mildred and thousands like her clinical governance needs to come out of the committee and boardrooms and into every care package.

The contracting framework of the internal market encouraged trusts to comply with the above elements. The development of PCGs and PCTs should produce a more systematic response to these issues in primary care.

Conclusion

Clinical and corporate governance processes, procedures, structures and approaches are all best seen as attempts to bolster the confidence that the community has in primary care and ensure that it is safe:

- for patients to put their lives in its hands
- for staff to develop their careers in the sector
- for the community and taxpayer to trust PCTs (and their equivalents elsewhere) to lead and direct the rest of the NHS, by controlling the vast majority of its resources as illustrated in Figure 3.4.

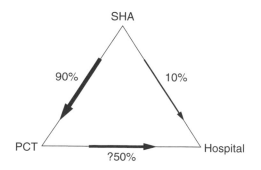

Figure 3.4:   Control of NHS resources by PCTs.

References

1 Cadbury Report (1992) *The Financial Aspects of Corporate Governance*. Gee Professional Publishing, London.
2 Ramsay J *et al.* (2000) General practice assessment survey (GPAS) 1998. *Fam Prac.* **17**: 372–9.
3 Department of Health (1997) *The New NHS: modern, dependable*. DoH White Paper, London.
4 European Commission (2001) *European governance*. A White Paper. Commission of the European Communities, Brussels.
5 European Commission (2001) Fritz W Scharpf, *Common concerns vs the challenge of diversity*. Jean Monet working paper 07/01. New York University School of Law.
6 Audit Commission (2001) *Hidden Talents*. Audit Commission, London.

CHAPTER 4

Primary care as a learning system

Introduction

This chapter takes us on a journey. The journey explores how the primary care sector might learn the lessons of previous chapters and adapt to the circumstances of the twenty-first century; might become fitter to deliver on its responsibilities as they evolve and change; and might grow and adapt to change. The chapter considers the factors which underpin effective learning and should equip us to use later chapters more effectively. Like many journeys this one has no definite end. We have to remember that life in the primary care sector is not precise, structured or clear cut; it is not simple – like Tom Lehrer's parody of the German rocket designer Werner von Braun, 'Once the rockets are up, who cares where they come down; that's not my department'. In the world of primary care it is not so simple to deny responsibility.

Context

The primary care sector has evolved as the first point of contact between individuals with perceived health needs and those charged with addressing those needs. As has been described by Barbara Starfield,[1] the sector in the United Kingdom is regarded internationally as being well developed and characterised by:

- its accessibility
- the continuity of care it offers
- the biographical nature of the care
- the undifferentiated nature of the care
- the holistic approach to synthesising physical, emotional, psychological and spiritual elements.

This all implies that the primary care sector is *reactive by design*. This means that:

- it reacts to what it is presented with
- it is non-judgemental
- it is free at the point of use
- it is unrationed

- it is almost sponge-like in its capacity to absorb whatever demands individuals and the community make on it.

If these have been the essential *design features* of the UK's primary care sector through the first 50 years of the NHS, then we at least need to ask the question whether they remain appropriate.

As the world around it changes, so the primary care sector needs to reflect on the significance of the changes to its own power, its responsibilities, its relationships and its behaviour. Then the sector has to learn the lessons and adapt to changing circumstances – otherwise it risks losing the confidence of the community. This is not to say that the heritage and enduring values of the sector should be thrown away – simply that failure to learn and adapt is risky.

This chapter will consider several aspects of primary care as a learning system. First, we will consider how some of the key design features are being challenged by modern circumstances and how relevant they remain as technology and society change. Then the chapter looks at how fit individuals and the whole sector are for the modern world, how adaptable, how responsive and how sensitive – this is examined using the Senge[2] disciplines, as a way of promoting 'constructive analysis' and hopefully opening up new insights supporting appropriate approaches to development.

Disease focused or *health* focused?

The major characteristics of the sector, e.g. accessibility, continuity, comprehensiveness, etc., were developed in an era when the sector's major responsibility was the management of acute and chronic disease. In the early 1950s, the sector faced annual epidemics of viral infection, the legacy of tuberculosis and chronic disease left over from the times before the NHS, and did so with a limited formulary of medicines and limited specialist support. As time has moved on, so the issues facing the sector have evolved to include health promotion and disease prevention as well as the continuing responsibility for disease management. Characteristics such as registration, continuity and biographical care make the sector an attractive option for any planned health promotion and disease prevention activity. However, there is an obvious conflict with open accessibility and being responsive to patient-initiated demand, especially when the capacity of the sector is challenged by high levels of demand, not always from those whose health needs are greatest.

Throughout the 1990s, the pressures on the primary care sector have become more and more concentrated on disease prevention, e.g. flu immunisation programmes, smoking cessation and screening services. These have rarely been implemented with adequate additional resources, have continually broadened the remit of the sector and have challenged the ability and capacity of staff to cope. The risk is clear – trying to do too many things may mean doing none of them well.

If the primary care sector is to effectively shoulder all of these responsibilities, which the community expects, then some reconsideration of the design features of the sector, or of its capacity may be needed.

The Wanless Report[3] has recommended a rapid, if incremental, approach to increasing the capacity of the primary care sector:

- additional clinical staff
- a major investment in information technology and management infrastructure
- modernisation or replacement of the entire estate over 10 years. A survey by the district valuer in 1998–99 suggested that:
  - nearly 80% of primary care premises are below the current recommended size. Only around 40% are purpose built. Almost half are either adapted residential buildings or converted shops and over 60% are over 30 years old
  - a fifth of the premises are in the private rented sector, almost two-thirds are owner occupied and the remainder are health centres, owned by NHS trusts or PCTs
  - although most surgeries are located within a quarter of a mile of a pharmacy, less than 5% are co-located with a pharmacy and around the same proportion are co-located with social services.

Overall the quality of the primary care estate and the range of services provided varies markedly from area to area. In particular, the most deprived areas tend to have the worst primary care facilities.

Current plans assume that two-thirds of the primary care estate will be upgraded or replaced by 2006, generally using private finance in line with current practice. The review has gone further by assuming that the entire primary care estate will have been modernised by 2010–11. To gauge the maximum cost and assuming that it costs on average £560 000 to replace a unit, the cost of upgrading or replacing all 10 500 primary care premises over the next decade would be £5.9bn, corresponding to an annual revenue cost of around £550m by 2010–11. This compares with a current figure of around £320m. We need to reflect that currently independent contractors are responsible for providing their own premises – by renting or ownership. Investment in premises forms a significant commitment for many – and through notional rent and cost rent schemes has, in the past, provided a useful retirement lump sum for contractors. The extent of the estate modernisation programme recommended by Wanless is likely to be beyond the resources of most independent contractors. It would seem likely that private sector corporate finance will be needed to meet his recommendations. We also need to reflect that by owning and capitalising premises, contractors, particularly GPs, have:

- had great difficulty moving between practices – even when such a move, or retirement, might have been in everyone's best interest

- sometimes suffered from negative equity and penalty charges when mortgages have to be transferred
- sometimes regarded non-property-owning partners and practices as 'second class' with consequent strain on relationships.

But this only addresses the structural design features – what of the attitudes, values and beliefs which are challenged by the changes in roles and responsibilities of the last decade and predicted for the future?

All of us, as individuals, have to react to change in personal circumstances. The ease with which we adapt and respond to the challenges which life throws at us varies a great deal from individual to individual. We know that the process can be challenging – the death of a close relative, moving house, losing one's job, etc. are all recognised as major life events which may cause personal and family distress and even depression. The more minor everyday challenges of raising children, balancing work and home, relationships at work and managing the family budget also constantly challenge each of us and force us to develop behaviour patterns which are able to respond and accept such challenges and adapt to them.

In considering how the primary care sector responds to the major challenges it faces, as well as the everyday issues that trouble it, it can be helpful to consider:

- several *aspects* which between them determine how the sector adapts
- several *perspectives* which illustrate how individuals view and respond to change
- several *dimensions* to responsiveness which can help illustrate the balance between adaptability and continuing ongoing virtues.

Personal care focus or community care?

Traditionally the primary ethical responsibility and concern of all practitioners in the sector has been to the individual patient or client although for some – such as health visitors – the emphasis on community development has been greater. Individual registration, personal and continuing care have all served to promote this core personal perspective. However, group practice, social mobility, team care and 'cover' arrangements have all reduced and challenged the concept. If personal and continuing care *really* matters, then PCTs will need to design in incentives to promote it.

The key tasks of PCGs and PCTs extend beyond providing personal care to assessing the health needs of the community, commissioning care and working in partnership with social services. Primary care organisations and practitioners need to reflect on the appropriateness of aspects of their heritage, the views or perspectives of the range of stakeholders involved and the dimensions to be considered in balancing the needs of individuals with health needs, against the needs of the broader community.

- Aspects of heritage
  - professional values
  - independent contractor capitalist
  - demand led
  - accessibility
  - registration.
- Perspectives or views of stakeholders (Figure 4.1)
- Dimensions (Figure 4.2)

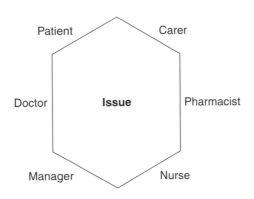

Figure 4.1:   The views or perspectives of stakeholders in primary care organisations.

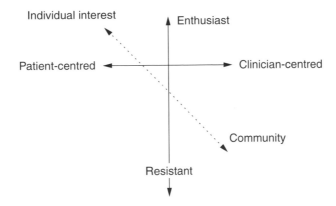

Figure 4.2:   Dimensions to be considered in balancing individuals' health needs with those of the wider community.

Figures 4.1 and 4.2 are by no means comprehensive – they are offered to help you build up your own balance sheet, to match your own personal approach to the past, the present and the future.

Understanding these issues can help those involved with planning the primary care sector and those who spend their working lives in the sector to be more in control of developments, be less threatened by change and make better decisions when faced with apparently conflicting choices. In order to promote such understanding, and therefore better decision making, further consideration needs to be given to some of the issues affecting individual, team, organisation and system behaviour. Understanding how the different elements making up the sector make decisions and respond to change is important if we are to view and develop the primary care system as a system which responds, adapts and learns from experience rather than one which confronts change with resistance, distrust and antagonism. The approach should be characterised by constructive debate and sustainable development as opposed to unhealthy scepticism and mouth curling cynicism.

Individual development

While all teams and organisations are made up of individuals, in the primary care sector the personal relationships with clients, which so many individuals have as part of their jobs, require particular attention for their own individual development. While it may be perfectly reasonable for large hierarchical organisations to concentrate their efforts on developing those few individuals who are vital to the delivery of key objectives, in the primary care sector quality of performance cannot be ensured by developing only key individuals because the sector has characteristics of:

- accessibility
- responsiveness
- non-hierarchical approach
- independent contractor directors
- long-term relationships
- personal and small organisational autonomy.

Rather, the planned development of *all* staff through a programme which matches their own needs with the organisation's needs and the sector's needs, is essential if the quality of care the sector provides is to be ensured.

- A core part of every individual development programme has to be attention to the motivation and personal development of every individual. Helping individuals to understand what motivates them, and to appreciate why they perform the way they do, how they are influenced by developments around them and how they are likely to react to changes affecting their career is perhaps the first place for any development plan to start. This understanding of self has, thus far, received very little attention in primary care educational programmes. Most clinicians and staff in this sector will have chosen to pursue their careers in primary care because they perceive that the balance between what they can offer and receive from their careers is complementary.

- Some will appreciate the flexibility of working hours that is available within the jigsaw of opportunities that the sector offers.
- Others will appreciate the long-term working relationships with colleagues and clients.
- Others, again, will particularly enjoy the large degree of clinical autonomy and independence which has historically been available.

Whatever the particular balance sheet any individual has, what counts is the extent to which the bottom line of that balance sheet continues to motivate the individual.

Committing primary care, as a sector, or as individual organisations such as PCTs, to supporting the learning of every individual within the organisation does not guarantee the quality of care within the sector, but without the commitment we can guarantee that the quality will not improve. As Kazoumo Inamori[4] has pointed out with reference to the commercial sector:

> Whether it is research and development, company management or any other aspect of business, the active force is 'people' and people have their own will, their own mind, their own way of thinking. If the employers themselves are not sufficiently motivated to challenge the goals of growth and technological development then there will simply be no growth, no gain in productivity and no technological development.

Tapping the potential of people, Innamory believes, will require new understanding of the subconscious mind, willpower and actions of the heart to form a sincere desire to save the world. This is even more relevant in primary care, and makes it imperative that the sector pays more attention to it. Individuals have to be encouraged to give up the old dogma of *control*, professional *arrogance* and *dependency* to reflect that the traditional patronising and paternalistic approaches to relationships are not designed to provide for individuals' 'higher order' needs for self-respect and self-actualisation. The ferment and conflict between antagonism and belligerence to change, and corporate development in the primary care sector will continue until organisations making up the sector begin to address these individual needs for every member of the workforce.

Investing in individuals' development is grounded in enhancing their individual competence and skills, but goes beyond it. It requires individuals to analyse themselves, their motives, their beliefs and their attitudes, i.e. what makes them tick. It means approaching their life as a creative work, not limited by nationality, creed, race, but part of the central force, which makes us human. The creativity is not limited to literature, sculpture or art but can be expressed through all aspects of life; it is as much to do with spirituality as it is with career and is as important for clerical staff as it is for clinical staff.

This process, or discipline[2] has become known as *personal mastery*. It requires us first to reflect and clarify what is important to us, what motivates us and what is the fuel from which our creativity springs. The second requirement for individual development is that we continually learn how to see what is going on around us with greater clarity and greater objectivity. Learning to gain control over events around us rather than constantly reacting to every new event as if it was happening in isolation; developing a clear picture of what is actually happening and where it is leading; having a clear perception or vision of where we are trying to get to – these all form parts of the creative energy which sustains this individual development. The energy has been known as *creative tension* – because individuals will constantly seek to balance the energy generated by motivation and learning against that energy consumed by reacting to patient and political demand. Creative tension can be destructive – the requirement for the future is to ensure that it is constructive.

'Learning' in this context does not mean acquiring more information but expanding the ability to produce the results and achieve the balance which all individuals strive for. It is a lifelong process of *generative* learning. If the primary care sector is to improve its performance incrementally it has to invest in this process of individual development.

Senge has described this investment as 'personal mastery' but this should not imply gaining dominance over people or things, rather mastery in this context means a special level of proficiency – think of a master craftsman or someone studying for a master's degree. Through their skill or mastery of the subject, higher quality emerges. Personal mastery suggests a special level of proficiency in every aspect of life – personal and professional.

The idea of individual vocation or calling has been important in the development of the caring professions and sectors for generations. For many individuals, their balance sheet will involve, to a greater or lesser extent, their 'calling' to care for the sick within the primary care sector. Sadly, the reality of careers can challenge such a calling unless it is seen as only one element in all individuals' balance sheets. The calling has to be seen as an element supporting personal development and growth, supporting the individual as part of their creative process and as fuel for the effectiveness and efficiency of the whole sector.

Individuals who have experienced this investment in personal development and have learned to understand themselves and to become more creative, will move on to become lifelong learners – they never arrive. Personal mastery is a process, a lifelong discipline. Individuals will become acutely aware of their inadequacies, the areas which they need to learn more about and grow through, and as a result of the analysis they will become more confident and more competent.

From the perspective of the PCT or of the whole sector, the motivation of individuals working within the sector, the degree of their commitment to their work and the sense of responsibility they have, will all contribute to enhancing the quality and effectiveness of care they provide. In addition, if individuals can find more personal fulfilment through their work, this will not only promote their own happiness but support the primary purpose of the sector in improving patients' lives and making patients and clients happier.

There will, of course, be resistance to this rather altruistic approach to individual development. Individuals and groups will resist the investment in individual development because of the challenge it poses to their own view and power base. In addition, one form of resistance is cynicism. Over-romanticising personal development can promote cynical comments about the extent to which it does not deal with skills, competencies and the 'real' issues which the sector faces. Convincing cynics means understanding them, their motivation and the mismatch between their own aspirations and achievements. The primary care sector has sadly abused many staff in the past, ruined many careers and damaged many individuals. Constant reorganisation, continuing subversion of an individual's career development to patient need and operational pressures, and continuing underinvestment in individual learning have left a cynical legacy. This legacy has to be challenged and overcome before the sector can release the creative energies described above.

As mentioned earlier, part of the resistance to individual development comes from *fear* and the *risk* that empowering people can be counter-productive. If the individuals within organisations do not share a vision of what they are trying to achieve, do not understand why empowerment matters and why individuals' and organisations' balance sheets need to complement each other, then empowering individuals will only create more stress and distress within the organisation. Investing in individual development can only be a part, one element, of developing the primary care sector. The commitment to developing individuals and personal mastery is naïve and foolish if the other elements of team and organisational growth, building a shared vision and looking at the system as a whole, are not considered as well.

In developing individuals as learners, the primary care sector and its leaders will need to understand the culture of the sector and its roles, responsibilities and relationships. Developing and expressing the following views are important elements in committing the sector to supporting individual development and learning from it.

- How the sector fits within the world.
- Reflecting on the underlying values and beliefs which have supported the sector's development.
- Expressing their vision and listening to others' visions of how they see the sector evolving.
- Learning from current realities.

The core strategy is to develop leadership role models. Leaders within the sector need to demonstrate their commitment to understanding themselves and to lifelong learning. They need to demonstrate through their actions and through their working lives their own commitment, otherwise the cynics will question their motives.

Mental models

As well as supporting individual growth and development, the primary care sector will need to balance the different perceptions and views of the world which individuals and groups within the sector hold. Developing the primary care sector through understanding these perspectives and working with them, rather than challenging them and trying to impose change on them, is much more likely to be successful. Individuals' perspectives or views of the world form part of their *mindset* or *mental model*. This is a multi-dimensional construct of how they as feeling individuals view the world, how it works, how it affects them and how they relate to it. Developing the primary care sector by understanding such mindsets, testing them and helping them learn from each other is likely to be more successful than denigrating or preferring particular aspects of each.

These mindsets are powerful for the following reasons.

- They are active – they shape how we act. If we accept people for what they are, we will act differently from if we believe people have to fulfil particular stereotypes. If I believe that I am basically shy and lack self-confidence and that my colleague is basically arrogant and self-opinionated, then this is likely to shape the way I behave and act within that relationship.
- They affect what we do. We respond to what we see and how we see it. We each of us observe selectively so that when we recollect a consultation, the individuals taking part will have experienced it differently and, as a result, while one may complain, the other may feel the consultation went well. This mismatch of perceptions or mindsets affects all aspects of our individual behaviour and how people react together.

It is not just individual mindsets or mental models that have to be considered, there are also team and organisational behaviour patterns and actions, which result from the collective mindsets involved. If a general practice 'believes' that patients are partners in delivering healthcare, then they are likely to act differently from a practice which believes that it is the provider of healthcare and patients the recipients. If a practice believes that it is in the business of promoting healthy lives, then it will act differently from one which believes it is in the business of caring for people with disease. If a pharmacy believes that it is in the business of boosting shareholders' value, it will act differently from a pharmacy which believes it is there to manage medicines effectively. If a nursing team believes it is there to promote the individual autonomy and happiness of patients referred to it, then it will act differently from a team who view their task as providing personal care and comfort for those same patients.

The problem with these approaches lies not in whether they are right or wrong – by definition each of these is a simplification or one-dimensional caricature of a complex picture. The problems arise because these views are tacit; they are not questioned, challenged, subjected to critical review and analysis. Because the perceptions remain tacit, they remain unchanged as the world around them changes and, while they may have been appropriate in the past, they may now be harmful. So, while the patronising paternalism of Dr Findlay may have been appropriate in rural Scotland at the start of the NHS, it may no longer be an appropriate perception for modern general practice in the post-family society. While nursing owes some of its perspectives to its origins through the Poor Law and Florence Nightingale, with the virtues of charitable giving and voluntary effort, and while health visiting has enjoyed the perspective of social education and advice in support of social change, such heritage and perspectives need to be challenged in the consumerist and post-industrial society in which we now live.

Failure to appreciate the importance of these different perspectives and the necessity of helping them evolve through analysis and challenge has been a problem in the primary care sector for many years. The very different approaches taken by different general practices, the different approaches to care taken by different branches of nursing, physiotherapy and occupational therapy have made teamworking and co-ordination of care across the sector problematic. Trying to develop a systematic approach to care within the sector, for instance in response to national service frameworks, is always going to be challenged when the individuals and groups within the sector have very different mindsets and perceptions about their roles and their responsibilities in the area under consideration.

Individuals' and groups' mental constraints or mindsets are often deeply held, cherished and held on to with an inertia which sometimes defies reason.

Box 4.1:   Repeat prescribing

To some extent, the repeat prescribing system in primary care is an example where each individual in the system behaves in a fixed or stereotypical way, be they:

- patients on regular medication
- clerical staff administering the system
- GPs authorising, controlling and directing the system as prescribers
- pharmacists dispensing the prescriptions and advising patients
- district nurses and carers supervising.

They know how to make the system work, they know their part in it and they don't question it.

The system has evolved to try to ensure the safe supply of effective medicines to those with long-term health problems needing continuing medication. However, the system has developed into a monster. It is an inefficient, time and energy consuming system which seems designed to ensure that everyone will be unhappy most of the time – patients and carers with the necessity to make unnecessary journeys and phone calls, clerical staff with ensuring the safe production of prescriptions, GPs with signing and checking hundreds of scripts each week and pharmacists with supervising the supply time and time again.

In the modern age, these inefficient and unnecessary systems designs have to evolve in a way which provides safe care efficiently – if supermarkets can supply fresh food efficiently, surely ...

In this example and in many other areas, the groups involved behave and relate to each other in an almost *tribal* way. While tribes, as a social construct, have much to commend them, they are not the most flexible, adaptable and responsive of groupings – they tend to fight each other rather than discuss, prefer marriage within the tribe rather than between tribes and are very territorial.

With the advent of new information systems and communication arrangements, the model of how a repeat prescribing system ought to work and who does what within it needs to be re-thought. But the energy, commitment and safety tied up in the current system – particularly the way community pharmacists are dependent on the volume of scripts for their income – means there is a considerable inertia to be overcome and it always seems easier to maintain the system rather than adapt it.

So if these perspectives and models can impede change, can freeze organisations and systems in outmoded practices, how can understanding them and working with them accelerate learning, improve performance and promote the quality of care provided? There are a few examples we can consider.

Using mindsets

Analysing and appreciating the perspectives of individuals and organisations is an important part of building a vision of what their future might look like. Over the last 30 years, a range of organisations have undertaken such analysis as part of *scenario planning*, as an aid to understanding how their organisation might develop in the future. Organisations as diverse as Royal Dutch Shell, The United Nations, the pharmaceutical industries and the NHS have realised that understanding the perspectives and mindsets involved can help them construct alternative visions of their future and through using them make better decisions about their own development.

The *Tomorrow's World* project similarly used these tools to consider the future of the primary care sector. www.radcliffe-oxford.com/challenge details two alternative pictures of how the primary care sector might look in a few years' time. These pictures have involved reflection on the roles of individuals and groups, their mindsets and perspectives and the challenges they face at present as part of the process of designing the future.

Another example, perhaps closer to primary care everyday reality, has been the kind of development 'away days' that practices and teams have been on in a rather random way.

Such developmental sessions have not only started the process of corporate development in primary care (sometimes), but they have also begun to challenge the individual and group mindsets and perspectives so as to develop some kind of a shared vision of what the organisation is trying to achieve. Developments such as participation in GP fundholding, locality commissioning, total purchasing and PMS have often resulted from such sessions.

Box 4.2:   Practice away day

Prestwood House Surgery had grown from nothing to looking after 6500 patients during the 1980s and 1990s. Following the ending of fundholding, the practice held an away day for the whole team in 2000 to consider how it would develop for the future. Following a process of small group analysis and discussion, the team agreed that a number of issues needed more attention than they had historically been given. These included:

- substance abuse
- the care provided in nursing and residential care homes
- teenage health
- chronic disease management including conditions such as epilepsy, diabetes, asthma and chronic bronchitis and osteoarthritis
- the supply of medicines
- the way the organisation is governed.

As a result of the away day, the practice agreed a PMS plus practice-based contract, with the LHA and PCG. Through this agreement, the practice accepted more responsibility for the above issues in exchange for security of funding for an agreed population and performance management arrangements to monitor progress and agree future developments. Over time, the move from a GP-governed organisation to an organisation reflecting the perspectives of all staff and patients has been initiated and while the process of transition will raise many questions about power sharing and challenges to individuals' and groups' perspectives, it is clear that the organisation is now much more responsive to change and more adaptable than it used to be.

The key skills involved in using the different mindsets and perspectives constructively as a set of tools in the primary care sector are:

- analysing the mindsets, understanding what they tell us about the attitudes and beliefs underpinning them and being able to interpret them in a way acceptable to those that hold them
- developing the necessary interpersonal skills to be able to work with individuals and groups in using their mindsets constructively.

In primary care, the consultation and interpersonal skills of practitioners are often well developed and appropriate for use in this area. However, the individual and group *defences* are also strong. These defences help protect practitioners and groups from the emotional pain caused by challenge to their identity and values and have to be respected if destructive behaviour is to be avoided.

Using scenarios

Scenarios, such as the two developed in the *Tomorrow's World* project (*see* www.radcliffe-oxford.com/challenge) can be used as a tool for understanding mindsets and perspectives. They force individuals and groups using them to consider how they would cope in different circumstances. This offsets the tendency we all have to imagine one particular future rather than the alternatives. When groups consider alternatives, they can begin to make choices, decisions and plans which take into account more determining factors and more predictable changes than they had previously. These are exactly the advantages that Shell enjoyed when it used scenarios to help it plan ahead and make decisions in the post-OPEC era of the 1970s.

Many groups, companies, services and nations have invested a great deal of time in understanding the perspectives/mindsets/mental models they work with and have found that, through this, they can change the way the organisation plans for its future. They have discovered that it is less important that they produce perfect plans than that they use the planning process, i.e. understanding perspectives and mental models, to encourage learning by individual teams and the organisation. Long-term success, in these terms, depends on the process through which teams change their shared mental model of their structure, the environment they are working in and their future. For this reason, the planning process and the learning process really become one and are perhaps best known as 'institutional learning'.

Large organisations, which have worked with mindsets as planning and learning tools over the years, have established systems and processes within the organisation to ensure that the analysis and use of the tools is safe for the individuals and effective in the organisation – just as confidentiality and 'Chatham House rules' have evolved in the health service. An example of the framework for using mental models is Hannover's Credo[2] on mental models.

Box 4.3:   Hannover's Credo on mental models

1   The effectiveness of a leader is related to the continual improvement of the leader's mental models.
2   Don't impose a favoured mental model on people. Mental models should lead to self-concluding decisions to work their best.
3   Self-concluding decisions result in deeper convictions and more effective implementation.
4   Better mental models enable owners to adjust to change in environment or circumstance.
5   Internal board members rarely need to make direct decisions. Instead, their role is to help the general manager by testing or adding to the GM's mental model.
6   Multiple mental models bring multiple perspectives to bear.
7   Groups add dynamics and knowledge beyond what one person can do alone.
8   The goal is not congruency among the group.
9   When the process works it leads to congruency.
10   A leader's worth is measured by their contribution to others' mental models.

Interpreting this for a PCT or one of its constituent organisations is possible, although of course it needs adapting to local circumstance. In particular, the role of leadership in the primary care sector is very different from that in a large corporation and we need to look at what is meant by 'internal board members'. These are, perhaps, best considered as the non-executive members of PCTs in that their role is to help executive managers and clinicians by testing or adding to the mental models/mindsets, thus promoting analysis. It should be noted that the goal is not congruency among the group of perspectives or trying to make everybody happy that their perspectives are really the same, but rather to value each for what it adds to the whole so that as the analysis and use of the perspectives proceeds, organisational, group and individual learning can occur.

The learning skills involved in analysing and using perspectives in this way are not new. The importance of *reflection* on learning in professions such as medicine has been known for a long time. While many professionals seem to stop learning as soon as they leave university, those who become lifelong learners become 'reflective practitioners'. The ability to reflect on one's thinking while acting, to learn from such reflective practice and to change one's actions are features which distinguish outstanding professionals who can move from being effective practitioners to becoming master practitioners. Phrases like 'thinking on your feet', 'keeping your wits about you' and 'learning by doing', suggest not only that we can think about doing, but that we can think about doing something while doing it.

The results of such reflective practice and of analysing perspectives can lead from simple linear step-by-step evolution of thinking, to quantum jumps or 'leaps of abstraction' where new ideas occur from the synthesis of reflection. This is another example of the kind of 'generative learning' which is required to move primary care from its past to its future. An example of this process working in practice is given in Box 4.4.

Box 4.4:   Leap of abstraction

'For the first 15 years I was a practitioner, I was always on duty on a Tuesday night and, in addition, was on duty every fourth weekend. These duties involved covering my practice list of 9000 patients and responding to emergency calls as appropriate. Over the years, the system became more effective as bleepers and mobile telephones were introduced and changes in IT enabled more information to be available to support decision making. Nevertheless, the out-of-hours burden was considerable for the practitioner and patients were often reluctant to call, even when they had pressing health needs. The introduction of commercial deputising services meant that some doctors were able to opt out of out-of-hours work but at considerable cost and as I was practising in a rural area, this was not an option for us.'

During the mid-1990s the development of GP out-of-hours co-operatives spread like wildfire across the country and transformed the out-of-hours commitment of general practitioners. This did not occur by any linear stepwise development of emergency cover within the practice but rather by a 'leap of abstraction' where thinking about out-of-hours cover for a population 'outside the box', enabled a new service to develop. Although not perfect, GP out-of-hours co-operatives have had a number of benefits.

- They have reduced the on-call commitment of most practitioners.
- They have encouraged development of more corporate and co-operative work between practitioners and practices.
- They have provided a more uniform and accessible service for patients.
- They offer an opportunity for the NHS to agree quality standards for out-of-hours provision.

As Senge[2] points out, 'Thinking about whole systems without understanding perspectives/mindsets/mental models, is like the DC3's radial air-cooled engine without wing flaps. Just as the Boeing 247's engineers had to downsize their engines because they lacked wing flaps, systems thinking without the discipline of mental models loses much of its power.' In other words, the two disciplines, using mindsets/mental models and systems thinking, are interdependent.

In the primary care sector, trying to design PCTs and considering their role as providers and commissioners of care, requires that they work with the mindsets of all those involved in the primary care sector or face drastically downsizing their expectations about improving efficiency in healthcare delivery.

Individuals in the primary care sector who realise the benefits of lifelong learning and personal mastery are less likely to have rigid and inflexible mindsets antagonistic to change and development. They will have challenged and changed their approach and should continue to push those responsible for the development of the sector to be more responsive to change in circumstance, more quality assured in its processes and more committed to the underpinning values of the sector.

As has been shown by John Sterman[5] most of our mindsets, or mental models, are systematically flawed. They are constructs of our own imagination and miss out on critical relationships, misjudge temporal relationships and often focus on variables that are most obvious or shout loudest rather than those which are most critical to development or success. Most of us do not see or take into account in our decision making the critical reinforcing feedbacks which help us to develop and grow when we are put under pressure. For example, can we learn and grow when we are threatened or challenged during a consultation? Understanding and learning from such flaws in our mindsets can be therapeutic.

Building commitment

While individuals will have their own mindsets and to a greater or lesser extent be masters of their own destiny, if they are to be more than a group of individuals and to contribute to the effectiveness of teams and organisations within the primary care sector, then their learning and mindsets have to be co-ordinated.

Co-ordinating the aspirations and activities of so many individuals with different skills, professional backgrounds, perspectives and values is not simple. Encouraging individuals to clarify their own personal vision of what they are try-ing to achieve, how they see their career and their work developing over future years and what they see as the opportunities for personal growth and development which might arise, can be a constructive way of helping groups of individuals, teams and organisations understand the common elements of their individual visions and appreciate the elements which they share rather than those which divide them. Using such an exercise to build the shared vision of the future of a team or organisation can be very energising for all the individuals concerned. If there is sufficient commonality of vision and if the individuals can come together around a shared collective commonality, i.e. if they can share a vision of what they are trying to achieve, then the energy and the drive produced can be many times greater than that available to any one person. This is the essence of syner-gistic teamworking which produces the synthesis of orchestral performance, the beauty of ballet, the dominance of Manchester United and the aura of the All Blacks. When the shared vision is towards long-term objectives and has a more spiritual dimension, then the production of cathedrals and the pyramids can be achieved.

What is required is for individual visions and perspectives to be understood, analysed, dissected and reformed in such a way that the individuals can all commit to the common, shared mindset or vision where individuals subsume their personal vision for the greater good. While one or more individual(s) may delineate the shared vision and describe it as part of gaining commitment, there is a danger that in doing so their own visions may predominate and contaminate the product. Shared vision cannot be imposed from outside although it will have external elements to it, i.e. making it fit for the external forces influencing it, as well as internal elements or housekeeping constituents which make it more comfortable for those who are members of the team or organisation.

We will all know examples of where adversity can produce effective teamworking for the common good. The Battle of Britain is often quoted as an example, but within the primary care sector, many will reflect on how effective teamworking can be in dealing with an epidemic, a terminal care situation or a major disaster such as a rail accident.

However, developing a shared vision and commitment to longer term objectives around a common view of what the primary care organisation and sector is trying to achieve, has been more problematic. The sector has rather been characterised by considerable variation in approach, values and commitment – but, nevertheless, there are some examples. At an individual level, consider the lengths to which couples with infertility problems will go in order to have a family; the sacrifice that parents will make for the sake of their children; and the long-term considerations involved in committing one's career to a GP partnership or the kind of district nursing contract which existed in the early years of the health service when marriage, family, holidays and personal property were not permitted.

Within any team or organisation, the extent to which any individual commits himself or herself will vary. This can range from complete commitment through to grudging compliance or even non-compliance and apathy. On the whole, a team will work better if individuals making it up are committed to it. But complete, unswerving, 100% commitment can be blinkering and there needs to be some questioning and challenge of the vision, as time passes, if the way is not to be lost. The speed limit in urban areas is 30 or 40 miles per hour, but anyone who is completely compliant and never exceeds this is unlikely to maintain the respect and acquiescence of all the passengers in their car. A teenager who always breaks the speed limit 'on principle' is equally unlikely to be popular with the police or his or her passengers. What is required is sufficient compliance and commitment but not to the extent of being totally unquestioning.

The relationship between the shared vision which a team, group of individuals and organisation commit to, and its *culture* is worthy of consideration. Consider recruitment of a new member of staff, be they clinician or administrator. How do they perceive the organisation or team they are considering joining? Aspects of the culture of the organisation such as whether it is welcoming, controlling or demeaning spring at least in part from the mindsets of the individuals making up the team and from the shared vision which they radiate when a newcomer comes over the horizon. Organisations with high staff turnover or which find difficulty recruiting, usually have these problems because of either a culture of disharmony and dissonance, or the lack of a shared vision with which any prospective new member can resonate.

Building shared vision is only part of developing teams and organisations. If the primary care sector is to be effective and the teams within it are to continue to evolve and improve the quality of care they provide, then the vision has to be further developed and given more depth by moving on to consider the underpinning values and beliefs which form the foundations on which that vision can be built. These governing principles describe the:

- 'what', i.e. the vision of what we want the world to look like or the purpose
- 'why', i.e. what the organisation is trying to achieve and why it has to be designed and operate in the way it does
- 'how', i.e. the agreement as to the route to be taken, the relationships to be developed and the rewards to be expected. By pursuing the shared vision further into these new dimensions, then the vision can become both more secure for the members of the team but also more resilient to the internal and external forces operating on it.

While the core values or attributes of the primary care sector have been well described,[1] the process in this chapter of understanding one's self, analysing mindsets and perspectives, integrating individuals' visions into a shared vision and appreciating the core underpinning values involved can make such common features of the system much more real. The extent to which continuity of care, biographical care, comprehensive and generalist care will remain attributes of the primary care sector and each organisation within it, will vary depending on the shared vision and values of the organisations making up the sector. While accessibility, i.e. first point of contact, is vital if patients/clients are to have faith in the sector, how such accessibility is managed will vary according to circumstances and from area to area.

Teams and team learning

Patient care and the maintenance of health has never been the sole responsibility of *individuals* in the primary care sector, even though *clinical responsibility* often rests with those individuals. The provision of care always demands the active participation of the recipient as well as the provider and, over time, a range of skills and perspectives are often needed to deal with a range of health problems which all of us experience in our lives. For many years, the concept of the primary health-care team has been promoted as a way of bringing together the perspectives and skills necessary to deal with the range of situations which individuals in the team face in their practising lives. These three elements, already discussed, are important for:

- understanding and mastering individual identities
- exploring and understanding the perspectives and mindsets of individuals
- bringing together these mindsets into building a shared vision or common understanding of what individuals are trying to achieve.

We need to reflect that a greater emphasis on group and team performance is required if the analysis of Michael West[6] is correct.

- There is much researched evidence, which suggests that, in some circumstances, teams may perform less effectively than individuals working alone. Personality factors, poor communication skills, individual dominance, status, hierarchy and gender, can all impede effective teamwork.
- The history of separate professional development in primary healthcare helps to explain why teamworking in this context has been relatively slow to develop. Research evidence suggests that although there are clear benefits from teamworking, there are many difficulties in primary healthcare which impede effective team functioning.
- Representatives in our research groups see great potential for teamworking in primary healthcare but suggest that fewer than one practice in fourteen is successful in building successful teamworking. They describe the main barriers as lack of shared premises; diverse lines of management; poor communications; lack of team meetings; professional elitism; GPs' independent contract status; power differentials; payment systems; and unresolved differences in orientation in the various agencies involved in primary healthcare. In particular, GP commitment to working in teams was seen as critical to team effectiveness.

The report reflects that clear structure and objectives in primary healthcare are essential if the context is to be provided within which co-operation and creativity can flourish and professionals can concentrate their energies on relieving suffering and improving the health and well-being of the population.

This analysis implies that the primary care sector needs to consider the design and functioning of the primary care team, the context within which it operates and the constraints on its effectiveness in more detail and in more depth if it is to be successful in delivering better quality care.

We will consider a few internal and external aspects of teams before concluding this section by considering the part they play in the *system*.

Teams can be considered as 'groups of people who need one another to act effectively'. They do this in the following ways.

- Making decisions. In primary care, individual practitioners' decisions might sometimes be better made as team decisions because of the implications they have for all the members of the team.

- Translating decisions into actions for the development of plans and the mutual support provided to members in implementing plans.
- Developing behaviour patterns, mindsets and visions, which help to translate the provision of care into defined organisational culture and learning.

Some of the ingredients to be considered include: alignment; discussion and dialogue; and practice.

Alignment

The greater the degree of alignment, the more powerful the impact. The alignment should go from (a) to (b) in the diagram below.

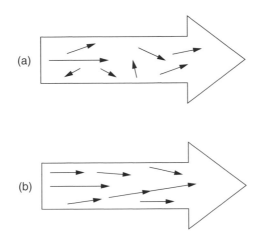

When a group of people function as a whole, we can consider them *aligned*. In most teams, the energies of individual members will often work at cross purposes as in (a). The fundamental characteristic of this relatively unaligned team is wasted energy. Individuals may work extraordinarily hard, but their efforts do not sufficiently translate into team output. By contrast, when a team becomes more aligned as in (b), a commonality of direction emerges and individual energies are more harmonised. There is less wasted energy. In fact, a resonance or synergy develops – their output is more coherent, like the light of laser as opposed to the light of a lightbulb or candle. There is a commonality of purpose, a shared vision, an understanding of how to complement one another's efforts. Individuals do not sacrifice their personal interest to the larger team vision; rather, their shared vision becomes an extension of their personal visions. In fact, alignment is the necessary condition before empowering the individual who can empower the whole team. Empowering the individual when there is a relatively low level of alignment worsens the chaos and makes managing the team even more difficult. In the primary care team, the multiplicity of employers, priorities and professional backgrounds makes alignment problematic.

Alignment produces commitment, both to each other and to the shared vision of the team. If an orchestra or jazz band is to *gel*, then the members need to be aligned and committed. Within an aligned team, there is a need for the members to think about complex issues quite deeply. This *analytical* and *critical* activity helps to cement alignment and build group identity. The team can then move on to agreed, innovative and co-ordinated activity to translate the results of their analysis into clear activity.

Box 4.5:   Building alignment

Prestwood House Surgery, as a result of its analytical work, decided to review the provision of care for teenagers. An evening meeting for all local teenager interest groups with over 50 participants was held. As a result, an innovative approach to teenage care has evolved with a reference group of stakeholders for the practice to work with in delivering new approaches to teenage health and disease management.

In addition, in a primary care team, members will be members of other teams as well. There is an ambassadorial function to promote team alignment in other teams and to spread best practice about innovation and coherence. New primary care organisations such as PCTs will have to challenge deeply embedded prejudices and institutionalised poor practice, where poor teamworking, disharmony and inefficiency prevent the development of high quality care. In challenging the past, the ambassadorial function where members from 'aligned' teams can spread the positive culture of coherence and quality enhancement can be constructive.

Discussion and dialogue

Discussion means talking together and *dialogue* means learning from each other. They are two of the essential processes through which teams can translate decisions into actions. They are both essential for effective teamworking. Discussion has the same derivation as percussion and concussion. It suggests a free flow of conversation during which issues may be analysed and dissected from many different perspectives provided by all those who take part. The purpose of the discussion is often to come to a consensus which then leads to a decision, leading on to an action. Sometimes, one individual's view may predominate but it may be modified or strengthened through discussion. A sustained emphasis on 'winning' is not compatible with giving top priority to alignment and coherence.

Bohm,[7] a quantum physicist, suggests that what is needed to bring about any change of priorities is dialogue, which is a different form of communication. Dialogue is derived from the Greek *dialogus*. *Dia* means through and *logus* means word or more broadly, the meaning. In dialogue, Bohm contends, a group accesses a larger 'pool of common meaning' which cannot be accessed individually.

The purpose of dialogue is to go beyond any one individual's understanding – it is a group activity where we are seeking synthesis of individuals' ideas to gain greater insight. We are looking for a common meaning where members of the team are no longer primarily in opposition nor can they be said to be simply interacting; rather they are participating in this pool of common meaning. In dialogue, a group explores complex, difficult issues from many points of view. Individuals suspend their assumptions, but they communicate their assumptions more freely. The result is a free exploration that brings to the surface the full depth of people's experience and thought and yet can move beyond their individual views.

Bohm identifies three basic conditions that are essential for dialogue to flourish.

1   Participants must suspend their assumptions. If an individual 'digs in his heels', the flow of dialogue is blocked. Suspending assumptions is a risky business but is essential if individuals are to open themselves up and become receptive to the exchange of ideas involved in dialogue.
2   All participants must regard one another as colleagues. Hierarchies and power blocks can inhibit dialogue. Members of the primary care team will come from different professional backgrounds or tribes and will each have their own mindsets, approaches to care and professional values. Respecting each other's professionalism, understanding the role that each plays within the team and within delivery care are important. All members have to respect and value each other as fellow team members if they are to learn from each other and, through dialogue, with each other.
3   Someone needs to 'hold the context' of dialogue. This can be an external facilitator but in teams experienced in dialogue – such as groups of elders in Indian tribes – then the context can be held within the team, either by one or more individuals. This is essential if constructive dialogue is to continue rather than be constantly diverted by defensive behaviour or distracted by comfort-seeking retreat into reminiscence or chit-chat.

If primary care teams are to learn together, then they will need to balance dialogue and discussion and through them a group or team identity will develop. Dialogue helps to develop a trust that carries over into discussions and through such discussions better decisions are made, more productive actions are planned and better care will be provided.

Sadly, membership of such teams is a risky business for individuals, particularly if they are insecure in their own identity and unsure of their own personal viewpoints. We all of us tend to retreat to defensive behaviour when challenged and this can prevent the kind of *team learning* which is required if teams are to move beyond symptomatic solutions to the problems they face, e.g. who will visit whom and what they will do, and move on to more systematic analysis and solutions such as empowerment and partnership.

Practice makes perfect

It cannot be stressed too much that team learning is a team skill. A group of talented individual learners will not necessarily produce a learning team, any more than a group of talented athletes will produce a great team. Learning teams have to learn how to perform together – an orchestra cannot just perform, it has to practise, as does a great football team.

In the primary care sector, teams will have worked together for some time and will have to break out from their historic ways of behaving together if they are to become more effective.

Donald Schon[8] described the essential principles of practice as experimentation in a *virtual world*. Use of the *Tomorrow's World* futures to help primary care teams consider how they would respond in the virtual world of the futures can provide this environment in which to practise. Through considering aspects of the two futures and the implications to members and teams as a whole, teams can move through discussion and dialogue to a greater coherence and synergy. The investment in such practice, away from the operational realities of day-to-day care is essential if primary care teams are to develop a deeper understanding and appreciation of each other's contribution and begin to learn together to produce 'team learning'.

Systems thinking

Bringing together the elements considered in this chapter is a necessary precursor to providing effective and efficient care.

- Understanding and mastering oneself.
- Working with individuals' perspectives, mindsets and mental models.
- Appreciating the value of visions and particularly building shared visions.
- Understanding and developing effective primary care teams and in particular promoting dialogue and learning as teams.

Each of the above disciplines on its own can help make the care provided by individuals and teams within the primary care sector more effective, but put together these disciplines can move the delivery of care away from being:

- *reactive* – simply responding to the demands of each patient in each particular situation, i.e. care of the sore throat or bad back
- *practitioner focused* – what the GP or physiotherapist or district nurse can contribute to the needs of a particular patient
- *short term* – what will deal with the presenting problem and keep the patient happy in the short term
- *comfortable* – what will promote safe and comfortable relationships between patients and staff

towards care that is:

- *proactive* – where care not only reacts to presenting problems but also guides behaviour towards prevention and improving health
- *team and partnership focused* – where care is partly the responsibility of the individual client/patient and partly that of the practitioners and administrators making up the primary care team with the individual practitioner's responsibility limited to his or her area of expertise
- *long term* – where the presenting issue or episode is seen as part of the biographical care of the patient and the long-term relationship that he or she will have with the primary care team, e.g. the sore throat in the teenager is part of the relationship which can discuss glandular fever as the 'kissing disease' and support discussion of relationships and family dynamics
- *challenging* – where the lifestyle and behaviour patterns of clients/patients can be challenged rather than colluded with. Pharmacists might challenge smokers' continual purchase of cough mixtures or mothers asking advice about coughs and colds in their children by challenging them to stop smoking, read and learn about how children become immune to viruses and support them in becoming more coping and caring parents and individuals.

Each of these transitions helps to support practitioners and primary care teams in moving from becoming simply responsive to the demands of clients/patients and seeing each item or episode of care as discrete episodes and towards a more systematic approach to the provision of care which complements the heritage of continuing, holistic, biographical family care which has so distinguished the heritage of the primary care sector from that of specialist hospital care. This *systems* approach will require primary care teams and organisations to understand some elements of complexity theory.[9]

The universal language of business is financial accounting, but accounting deals with details or items, rather than *dynamic complexity*. It offers snapshots of the financial condition or status of business but does not describe how those conditions were created. Today, there are several tools and frameworks that provide alternatives to traditional financial accounting as a language. These include competitive analysis, 'total quality' and scenario methods, such as scenario planning. None of these tools deals with dynamic complexity very well – but the use of system archetypes and an appreciation of paradigms can be helpful in understanding how systems thinking, or the physiology of the primary care sector, works. This is the agenda for the next chapter – bringing together the learning disciplines of this chapter with the analysis of systems to provide a framework for understanding the *physiology* or dynamic complexity of the primary care system rather than just its *anatomy* or structure.

Conclusion

Primary care practitioners, the teams they work within and the organisations they are part of have been adapting and evolving to the changing world in a rather random way. Using the approach described in this chapter, to encourage development in a more coherent, balanced and constructive way will help PCTs and the whole sector demonstrate that the responsibilities they have shouldered are appropriate and safe, the community can trust the sector and the sector can be secure in its own identity.

References

1 Starfield B (1994) Is primary care essential? *Lancet.* **344**: 1129–33.
2 Senge PM (1993) *The Fifth Discipline. Business.* Random House Books, New York.
3 Wanless D (2002) *Securing Our Future Health: taking a long-term view.* HM Treasury, London. http://www.hm-treasury.gov.uk/wanless
4 Inamori K (1985) The perfect company: goal for productivity. Speech given at Western Reserve University, 5 June 1985.
5 Steerman J (1987) Misperceptions of feedback in dynamic decision making. MIT Sloan School of Management Working Paper WP-1993-87. Cambridge, MA.
6 West M and Slater J (1996) *Team Working in Primary Health Care. A review of its effectiveness.* HEA, London.
7 Bohm D (1965) *The Special Theory of Relativity.* WA Benjamin, New York.
8 Schon D (1983) *The Reflective Practitioner: how professionals think in action.* Basic Books, New York.
9 *BMJ.* (2001) **323**: 625–8, 685–8, 746–9, 799–803.

CHAPTER 5

Systems thinking in primary care

Warning: This chapter is quite complex, assertive and often challenging. It deliberately contains many unsubstantiated arguments so as to provoke the reader.

Introduction

While the previous chapter explored the elements, which together can promote a culture of learning and development in primary care, this chapter looks at *systems thinking*[1] as applied to primary care and explores some of the *design features* of primary care which affect its ability to learn, develop and deliver better care.

Systems thinking (ST) is an approach to viewing or focusing on the whole process rather than individual bits – looking at films rather than still pictures and plays rather than individual scenes. Figure 5.1 illustrates this. The whole diagram is the 'system' containing several 'subunits', 'archetypes' and 'orbits' or 'paradigms'. Systems thinking requires us to put together all the elements making up the system, so as to understand how they relate to each other and to appreciate the principles underpinning the system's performance.

To help us explore ST in the NHS primary care system we will use two analytical tools:

- understanding *paradigms*
- recognising *archetypes*.

But first we have to establish the difference between the primary care *sector* and the primary care *system*.

The primary care sector is that part of the welfare sector to which citizens have direct, first point of contact, access (*see* Figure 5.2).[2]

The primary care system refers to the design of the sector:

- how it is put together
- how it works
- how it delivers care
- how it is managed
- how its internal and external relationships are organised
- how it learns and develops over time.

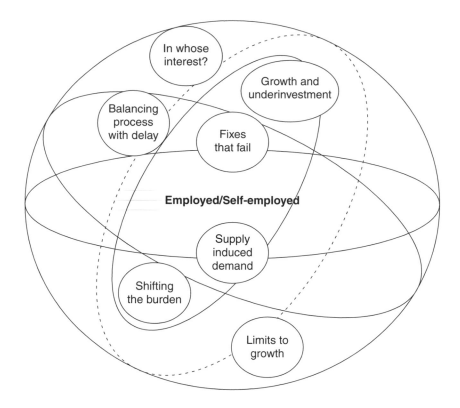

Figure 5.1:   Primary care paradigms and archetypes.

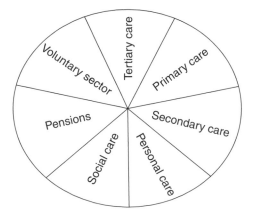

Figure 5.2:   The healthcare sector of the welfare sector.

This means looking at the context within which individuals and teams working in the sector operate and work together. It means looking at the *attitudes, values* and *beliefs* held within primary care, and also at some of the forces which shape practitioners and other stakeholders as individuals and teams and how they are responding to the pressures they have to cope with.

To understand paradigms and archetypes we again need to define what we mean:

- **Paradigms** are patterns or models which describe how the system is put together. If we look at Figure 5.1 as the primary care system, then its paradigms are descriptions of the design features which characterise it – the patterns which describe it and the models or approaches that influence its performance.
- **Archetypes** are *recurring themes* which we can learn to recognise. They:
  - underpin how all systems work
  - describe and determine how the system will respond
  - require us to shift our approach from one which thinks structurally to one which thinks *dynamically*
  - help us understand and interpret why any system works the way it does
  - fundamentally help us appreciate that systems work the way they do because that is how they are *designed* to work.

An analogy from the education sector can help to illustrate the use of the terms *system, sector, paradigm* and *archetype* as well as the importance of attitudes, values and beliefs in determining performance.

Box 5.1

Helen was starting a secondary school. She felt well prepared, she was happy and contented and had done well at her primary school and was going to the new school with many of her friends and a glowing report from her primary school headmistress. She knew the way to school, had visited it for a day, had read about the school on its website and was keen to grasp the opportunities, which she knew were lying ahead.

What she did not realise was the extent to which the institution of a large secondary school was going to affect her learning. The way in which disruptive children and overburdened teachers would make it difficult for her to learn and the isolation and feeling of floundering that she was going to feel in a school which was some 10 times larger than her primary school. She did not realise how pressurised her time was going to be, how much she was going to have to fit into and mould herself around the routine of school and homework, and the extent to which her success would be down to that spark of motivation and enthusiasm which she might or might not find.

In this analogy from the education *sector*, the comprehensive *paradigm* is dominant in the secondary education *system*. The archetypes Helen will experience, and which will hopefully enhance her learning include the following:

- *Shifting the burden to the intervener.* The task of the school is to support Helen's learning rather than take a 'chalk and talk' approach to teaching her, or 'ram down her throat' what she needs to know. This is the shift to supporting student centred learning – a shift in the locus of power from the provider to the recipient.
- *Escalation.* In the classroom context this so often leads to detention and conflict, to victimisation and bullying, but it can also lead to sporting excellence, scholarship and leadership. One thing leads to another in either a vicious or a virtuous cycle.

How these and other archetypes impact on Helen's development will be fundamentally affected by the *attitudes* of Helen's family and school to her education and development and her own attitude to the school; the *values* which underpin their relationships and culture; and the *beliefs* they all have about the purpose of education and its place in society.

This chapter then looks at some of the design features of the primary care system (analogous to Helen's new secondary school) in the British NHS or system (analogous to the education system) and particularly those which determine both the patients' experience of care within the sector and the staff's attitude to working within primary care. To do this, we are going to look at the sector in two different ways: by considering the paradigms describing aspects of the system and the archetypes determining how it behaves.

Although considered separately, both archetypes and paradigms, along with the elements of the previous chapter when put together, begin to describe the physiology, or inter-relating forces, which determine the quality and success of care provided within the sector. While we can, and will, consider individual paradigms and archetypes, and give illustrative examples of each, these are inevitably biased by the author's background and perspective. Readers will need to reflect on their own experience if they are to get the most out of this analysis.

Paradigms

The overarching design of health systems in different countries marks their 'top level' paradigm.

1   The NHS is state funded, free at the point of use and available to all, providing a **total care** system from the 'cradle to the grave'.[3]
2   This is in contrast to the **free market** paradigm of healthcare organisation in the USA which relies on personal funding, as opposed to state funding and only covers a proportion of the population.

3 A **'mixed system'** paradigm which applies in many western European countries, where individuals fund part of the system and the state the rest.

In the NHS, state funding and control implies a cohesive but centralised approach to determining *what* care will be delivered and *how* it will be delivered. Also what the roles, responsibilities and relationships between the system and the end user will involve.

Within the NHS paradigm, certain features are worthy of comment because they affect how the system works.

1 'Free at the point of use' means that to a greater extent than in most other health systems, care is provided to the individual without the cost of that care being an immediate concern. While this might be the altruistic approach, it would be naïve to think that the funder of this system – in this case the tax-payer – would not have an interest in ensuring cost effectiveness. Neverthe-less, it has been important in freeing the individual consultation from the issue of payment and has stopped those needing care from refusing to seek it because of their inability to pay.
2 The NHS paradigm has meant a more cohesive approach to public health problems, such as HIV, CJD, cancer screening and care of the elderly[2] than has been possible in other systems.
3 The NHS paradigm has produced a fairer system where everybody in the population has equal access to care, even if at times it feels as if this has been at the expense of quality. In the NHS, quality assurance has been less developed than in insurance or 'end user' (citizen) funded systems where 'he who pays the piper (the payer), calls the tune' means a greater incentive for quality assurance.

The Labour government's first health white paper, *The New NHS: modern, dependable*[4] introduced a much more corporate approach to the development of the primary care sector. For the first time, independent contractors and their organisations were to become part of larger, more corporate, organisations. Contractors and other healthcare professionals were to have considerable power and influence over the development of these organisations but for the first time this was to be balanced by their boards of directors which also included lay and social services representation alongside general and financial management expertise. Primary care groups, and their equivalents in Scotland, Wales and Northern Ireland, have evolved rapidly in response to political pressure towards becoming autonomous PCTs. These bodies have additional attributes of corporate organisations, such as the employment of staff, the ownership of premises, and the provision of care as well as the commissioning of specialist services. The extent to which they succeed in fostering the development of effective primary care services through independent contractors, while at the same time encouraging corporate approaches to governance, gatekeeping and clinical quality will be a major factor in determining their success. The extent to which independent contractors are prepared to act corporately in response to the establishment of PCTs will undoubtedly vary and it will be some years before we can see whether this experiment has been successful.

Major development in the primary care sector, in terms of human resources, capital and revenue spending, has to be safe or the Treasury, as the funder of the sector, will not trust the sector. If that happens then the 'experiment' of developing a primary care led service will fail. The deal on offer would seem to be new investment in exchange for the development of more trustworthy governing arrangements including a more corporate approach to the provision and commissioning of care.

Paradigms then are models or patterns; essentially patterns which are made up of elements which, between them, form a cohesive whole. In different situations or countries, the local circumstances will influence the design of the system and alter the paradigms. The communist system in Eastern Europe and Russia produced a paradigm characterised by economic stagnation, overburdened centralised bureaucracy, lack of incentives for entrepreneurship, high investment in education, 'exemplar projects' such as space exploration and dictatorship. The forces, which led to the dismantling of the Berlin Wall and the fall of communism, led to a 'paradigm shift' away from the communist system and towards democracy. It is useful to remember this example because it illustrates the following points.

- That the paradigm or model has a number of features which distinguish it and which are inter-linked or consequential from each other, and which make up an inter-related system with the elements being dependent on each other – just like a physiological system with feedback loops, homeostasis or balancing mechanisms to maintain the status quo.
- That paradigms are influenced by external forces which subtly alter the relationship between the elements and the whole physiology of the system. As a result, in the end, a critical point is reached where the whole paradigm becomes less 'fit for purpose' and shifts in such a way as to be more adaptable and better suited to the change in circumstance.
- There are a range of forces which combine to influence paradigms and it is useful at this stage to think of them under a number of headings, although they are not mutually exclusive and certainly do not describe all the influences which can produce change.

Political forces

The anti-apartheid movement and the African National Council in South Africa challenged and eventually produced a paradigm shift in the political system in South Africa away from the apartheid of the 1990s. Here we have a political force – the will of the majority – changing the whole political system despite an absence of control over the levers of power, military muscle or wealth.

Economic forces

The rise of Nazism in Germany in the 1930s can be considered as having been promoted by economic deprivation following the First World War and similarly the success of Thatcherism in the UK throughout the 1980s was determined by the economics of market forces and individualism.

Social forces

The changing patterns of family life in the UK towards a post-family society, serial monogamy, an elderly population, late parenting, fragmented and migrant communities and multiple careers are all social trends which influence many of the systems in the country such as education, law and order, housing and leisure as well as health.

Technological forces

Whereas the above are all relatively 'slow fuses', i.e. they are forces which act over long periods of time, gradually building up until they force a paradigm shift, technological forces can act much more quickly. The introduction of television and telephones rapidly changed communications, but compared to the Internet, mobile phones and antibiotics were relatively slow to influence health service paradigms. New technologies can change many of the ground rules underpinning the way the system works almost overnight. The introduction of fibre optic technology, enabling endoscopic diagnosis and surgery; the launch of new drugs such as H2 blockers and neuroleptics; the establishment of new materials such as plastic disposable syringes, PVC window frames and nylon tights have all produced much more rapid, but sometimes less fundamental, changes in paradigms.

While these forces all combine to change the way systems work, they do not necessarily produce the same change in the way individuals feel – in their *values, attitudes* and *beliefs*. Individuals vary in the degree to which they are keen, able and willing to adapt to changes in the forces and paradigms. Their individual success or failure is largely determined by the extent to which they are able to respond to and harness the forces, always remembering that while some may be offering great potential for improving the system, others may be a seven day wonder. A little caution is always wise – think of Betamax videos, Thalidomide, Osmosin and the Sinclair C5 as examples. We have to reflect that individuals' values, attitudes and beliefs have been moulded through their life as a result of their experiences, their culture and background, their professional identity and heritage and the other parts of their life, for example family responsibilities and outside interests.

With the above in mind, we will now look at a number of the other paradigms involved in the delivery and organisation of healthcare within the NHS. Although described individually as *whole service paradigms, professional paradigms* and *sector paradigms*, we need to remember that they are all inter-related and influenced by the above forces. Breaking them down in this way is useful to help us understand the way the systems are working and useful to help us understand how forces are operating on them, but nevertheless, we have to realise that such a description is too 'two dimensional' and 'anatomical', whereas in real life these issues are at least three dimensional and physiological rather than anatomical. Thus, the relationship between the elements of the system is at least as important as the description of the elements themselves and there are always more than one or two perspectives to be considered in interpreting and understanding how the system works. Thus in the description of the comprehensive paradigm in the secondary education system the relationship between Helen, her parents and the school is as important as the school itself and there will be a range of views about how well the system is working for Helen.

Whole health service paradigms

If we return to look at the healthcare systems of different countries, then we can begin to describe them by considering the extent to which the systems are either funded by individual service users at the time they are using the system or through personal contributions to an insurance fund or alternatively funded centrally by the community. This can be considered as one dimension (*see* Figure 5.3).

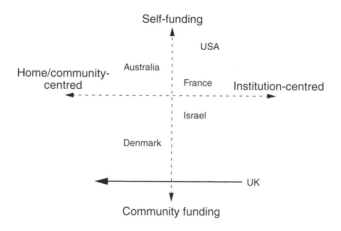

Figure 5.3: Whole health service paradigms.

In addition to this, we can look at systems in different countries and consider the extent to which they are either oriented towards care in the home setting, or, alternatively, oriented towards care in hospital or institutional settings. Figure 5.1 illustrates how the systems in different countries can be separated on such a diagram and we can then go on to look at how the forces operating on the system are moving the service, e.g. see how the UK has moved/is moving away from an institution-centred position.

The reasons why the UK paradigm is becoming less institutionalised can be examined under a number of headings.

- *Political.* In a centrally directed, politically driven service, institutional care may be seen as only bringing more problems – trolley waits, waiting lists, etc., while home based care is more patient centred, less risky for the politician and less of a financial 'black hole'.
- *Economic.* Less capital intensive care means more resources available for personal care and less reliance on buildings. In a country whose estate is decaying, the attraction of care outside hospital with less need for capital investment is obvious, but remember the Wanless Report (*see* Chapter 4).
- *Sociological.* Institutional care is depersonalising and promotes a culture of dependency. Home based care strengthens community and family networks and challenges the dominance of professional models which are so dominant in hospitals.
- *Technological.* Fibre optics and microprocessors, telecommunications and therapeutics – all permit and drive care away from institutional settings. While in highly technocratic, market driven societies such as the United States of America, high-tech institutional care may be promoted, in the UK such tendencies are resisted because of their cost and the difficulties involved in implementing radical changes in clinical practice in a system without effective clinical leadership.

Primary care paradigm

If the above considerations about whole health service paradigms seek to compare services between countries, then our examination of the primary care paradigms in the UK will reflect that there are many elements of the primary care system which are unique to the UK and we will not seek to compare the UK primary care system with other countries. Rather, we will look at how the primary care sector within the UK is changing, how the paradigms underpinning the design of the sector during the first half century of the NHS are being influenced by the forces acting on it and how the pattern of primary care – or the paradigm of primary care as a sector – is evolving. We shall follow this by looking at some of the professional paradigms involved and some of the sector paradigms, particularly from a primary care perspective.

Figure 5.4 illustrates two dimensions of the primary care paradigm – but of course there are others.

If we look at the system or sector of primary care over the last 50 years, we can see how care provided by individual practitioners working either in isolation or 'side by side' within a 'fragmented' governance framework, i.e a framework which is made up of highly independent subunits with little or no integration

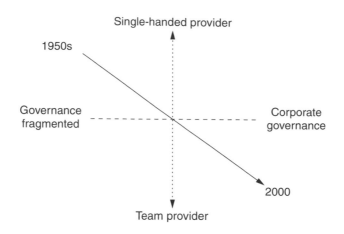

Figure 5.4:   Primary care paradigms.

between them, has been evolving towards a more corporate framework delivered through more cohesive care teams. The forces which have been operating to change or shift the paradigm of primary care away from the 1950s fragmented paradigm and towards the corporate primary care trust paradigm can be summarised as follows.

- *Political.* The need for the sector to be more responsive to the views of the community, its priorities and its concerns about performance, decision making and power. In addition, the desire for change or 'modernisation' is a reflection of the political view that the sector has been slow to adapt to the changing world and less than responsive to political imperatives.
- *Economic.* With more and more care being provided in the primary care sector, so the proportion of NHS resources, which are consumed within the sector, has increased. The requirement for the sector to demonstrate that it provides value for money, that investment in the sector is safe and that the sector can use resources efficiently has increased as a result. As the NHS has struggled to find enough money to fund the secondary and specialist care sectors, so the requirement for a less capital intensive solution to providing modern healthcare has increased. The provision of capital by independent contractors has been allowed relatively free reign, but now the need is to plan for increased capital expenditure, independent contractors cannot be relied on to provide it in response to the communities' priorities, and *corporate* PCTs will need to bridge the gap.
- *Sociological.* With social mobility increasing, the likelihood that any individual will know the primary care provider they are consulting decreases. In the past it was not uncommon for an individual pharmacist, doctor or nurse to know three or four generations of the family, but this is changing. While this biographical or long-term relationship based care remains an important

feature of general practice and the primary care sector, it is perhaps less of a dominant force than it was some years ago. In addition, universal education, change in family structures and consumerism are driving the primary care sector to be more responsive and less paternalistic than in previous years.

- *Technological* developments also significantly affect how the primary care sector is designed. While telephones enabled easier communications in the 1950s, nowadays it is e-mail and the Internet, mobile phones, etc. which make care more accessible and the need for interpretation of information more important. In addition, technological innovation through pharmaceuticals and health service technology has fuelled the increase of provider responsibilities that the sector has had to respond to, and the increase in the proportion of health service resources which it now has to account for.

As a result of these forces, the fragmented 1950s paradigm of the primary care sector is shifting. It is shifting so that it becomes more team oriented with the individual citizen's relationship with the sector being less personal. The paradigm is also shifting so that the governing arrangements within the sector are more corporate, and therefore more easily influenced by the community's priorities, and more open to scrutiny by the taxpayer. Inevitably, this can be seen as weakening the patient advocacy role of individual practitioners; the importance of registration and personal responsibility are also less dominant. While many practitioners and older patients will regret these changes in emphasis, they are the result of the rise of individual autonomy throughout the community and of increasing social mobility. While advocacy, etc. remains important for the weak and vulnerable and in circumstances where disease leads to dependency, it can no longer dominate the whole design of the primary care sector and therefore has become a less vital determinant of the primary care paradigm.

Professional paradigms

One of the key characteristics of the primary care sector throughout the first half century of the NHS has been the extent to which the professions involved in providing care within the sector have been dominant. As has been mentioned above, there are now a range of forces which are challenging this professional power base. We need to examine some aspects of the professional paradigms involved if we are to appreciate why they are responding the way they are and what the future might hold for them.

There are many professions involved in providing care within the primary care sector. Many of them have long and honourable heritages (*see* Chapter 1), but just as with the whole healthcare system paradigm and the primary care sector paradigm, so the professional paradigms can be reviewed by considering them against at least two dimensions.

Figure 5.5 separates the professional paradigms on the following bases.

1   The relationships between, and with, other colleagues; i.e. either operating
    with a great degree of autonomy as a 'loner' or operating with much more
    collective responsibility as a 'cohesive team'.
2   The other dimension considered in Figure 5.5 looks at the degree of depend-
    ency that characterises the relationship between the customer/client/patient/
    service user and the professional, as opposed to the extent of any promotion
    of patient autonomy which characterises the professional culture concerned.
    Of course, the position of any one profession within this diagram is variable
    depending on circumstance and to that extent the positions are somewhat
    arbitrary. Nevertheless, occupational therapists, smoking cessation advisers and
    counsellors all tend to see their primary purpose as promoting patient auton-
    omy while the heritage of nursing, community pharmacy and medicine has
    been much more centred around concepts of care and dependency with the
    emphasis on what the carer can do for the patient, rather than what the
    patient can do for themselves.

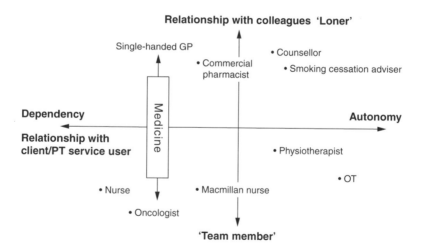

Figure 5.5:   Professional paradigms.

In particular, the 'medical model' or paradigm has been a dominant force within
the primary care sector for the first 50 years of the NHS. The particular
characteristics of the medical model which have been so dominant have resulted
from the following factors.

•   *Medical training* – equips doctors to understand pathology and to treat it.
    Unlike nurses, pharmacists, etc., doctors' training has equipped them to take
    personal responsibility for the management of the whole range of diseases
    which individuals may suffer from. Their postgraduate training through a

variety of specialities as well as time spent working with an experienced primary care doctor (as a GP registrar) has provided them with an apprenticeship model of training where their role as a diagnoser and manager of pathology has been dominant. The emphasis has been on diagnosis and management rather than on primary or secondary prevention of pathology, or complications, and has not provided incentives for patients to look after themselves, to refrain from pathology-inducing habits and behaviour, or to be responsible for their own health. While this model has many attractions, particularly when knowledge about pathology and diagnosis was limited, it may no longer be appropriate in an age where health promotion and disease prevention are increasingly important. This aspect of the model now needs to respond to the changing forces released by universal education, new technology, social change, etc.

- *Registration and capitation* – power within the primary care sector came partly from professional knowledge and partly from control over resources. Patients registering with a GP meant that all the health service payments, consequent on registration, followed – forming part of the power base of the individual GP. These arrangements have not applied to pharmacy, nursing, OT, etc., but have determined the distribution of the major funding stream (GMS) within the primary care sector. Through these capitation fees and registration arrangements, GPs employ staff, provide premises and run their own organisations. As discussed elsewhere, the registration system and associated payments form the foundation of the GP payment system and do not always encourage investment and service development, based on the health needs of the community. The caring values, the patient centredness, which attracted so many GPs to the speciality have to contend with the issue of profitability and business inherent in the registration issue.

- *Continuity of care*. GPs are required to provide care 24 hours a day, 7 days a week, 365 days a year, either personally or by arranging cover with other practitioners. This has provided every individual within the community with continual access to medical expertise within the primary care sector, which is not available in other countries or to other professions in the UK, e.g. pharmacy, OT, counsellors, dentists, solicitors, accountants, etc. It is not surprising, therefore, that primary care physicians (especially GPs) are regarded as a core feature of the primary care paradigm. Nevertheless, such primary care physicians are expensive to train, and as the proportion of care provided in primary care has expanded so it has become ever more important to ensure that this scarce resource is used efficiently. The concept of skill substitution, i.e. nurses doing some of the tasks which previously doctors did, and healthcare assistants doing some of the tasks that nurses historically did, has taken root. NHS Direct, walk-in centres and emergency care centres can be seen as a challenge to the continuity of care previously provided by GPs and to the dominance of the medical model. Nevertheless, these centres are largely organised and run based on essentially medical professional values, being interested in diagnosis and management rather than the traditional nursing role and values of care and support. What seems to be developing is the requirement for nurses to take on diagnosis, personal advice and care management responsibilities, but thus far, the training of nurses for such responsibilities has not been as rigorous as for GPs.

- *Prescribing.* As well as diagnosing and acting as personal advisers to their patients, GPs have been responsible for almost all prescribing in the primary care sector. As the costs of drugs have risen and the proportion of primary care budgets consumed by prescribing has risen, so the importance of this area to the power of the medical model has increased. Understanding therapeutics, managing medicines and, in particular, repeat prescribing systems which account for the majority of the costs involved, is a very important issue for everyone involved in the primary care sector. The degree of accountability that individual GPs have had for their prescribing behaviour has been limited in the past and has been a constant source of tension between them and the rest of the health service. Nevertheless, they are relatively cost effective prescribers compared to their colleagues in other countries.

  The move to supply more medicines without prescription (prescription only medicines to pharmacy supply) under the guidance of pharmacists and to introduce nurse prescribing, and, following the Crown Report,[6] the concept of dependent and independent prescribing can be seen as challenging the degree of control that GPs have over prescribing. There are, however, risks: other prescribers will have had limited training in management of medicines, diagnosis and pathology and the expectation that they will be more cost efficient than GPs may be confounded.

- *Gatekeeping.* GPs have been the sole gatekeeper to a variety of resources both within the primary care sector and outside it. Almost all referrals to specialist care have been channelled through GPs and they have also acted as gatekeeper to a range of social security, employment and certification services. The gatekeeper role has been seen internationally as an important contributing factor to the cost effectiveness of the NHS but has concentrated power in the hands of the GP to an extent which may no longer be sustainable as patients' individual freedom of choice, autonomy and mobility have made them less tolerant of 'gatekeeping'. Even with effective gatekeeping, the UK has some of the longest waiting lists and waiting times for specialist care; it has among the worst morbidity rates in the developed world for diseases such as coronary heart disease and cancer; and abuse of social benefits is as prevalent in the UK with its GP gatekeeping function as it is in other countries.

All of these issues affect the power of the medical model and the same kind of analysis could be undertaken for most of the other professions involved in the primary care sector. The extent to which any of the professional paradigms is adapting to the political, economic, social and technological forces operating on the primary care system is variable. Nevertheless, the forces are driving change and the professional paradigms will adapt just as apartheid, Nazism and communism have adapted.

Sector paradigms

The patterns or models of care provided in different sectors should also be considered as paradigms. Just as the primary care system contains a number of paradigms within it, so each of the other sectors – secondary, voluntary, social, etc. – contains paradigms which merit consideration. There are many including the following:

- emergency care
- health promotion
- elective care
- chronic disease management
- rehabilitation
- reproductive care
- dental care
- eye care.

As examples, we will look at the emergency care and dental care sector paradigms but the same type of analysis could be carried out for any of them and can be helpful if we are trying to understand why and how they are changing, why they need to change and how they might evolve for the future.

Emergency care

In this paradigm (*see* Figure 5.6) we can separate countries on the basis of the extent to which the emergency care systems are capitalised and the extent to which they are founded on a tradition of care at home or are centred around care in hospitals. The Third World countries such as Bangladesh and those in Eastern Europe have less capital intensive systems while the UK and USA differ in the extent to which they are focused on the home care setting or the hospital setting. Within the emergency care system, the extent to which diagnosis and management takes place in the home, in the ambulance, in the emergency room of the hospital or in a specialist unit, such as coronary care unit, will vary and technological and economic factors will drive change as in our other examples. Nevertheless, the case of thrombolysis and its introduction into the primary care sector in the UK can help to illustrate some of the difficulties. Thrombolysis needs to be given to people suffering a heart attack as soon as possible after symptoms occur. The drugs are relatively expensive and, at least initially, required considerable doctor intervention and time to administer. Health authorities found it easier to monitor thrombolysis given in hospital than in primary care as they had formal contracting arrangements which could be used to audit the quality of

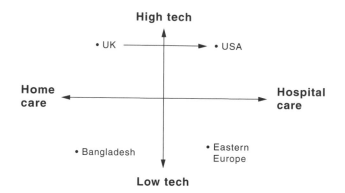

Figure 5.6: Emergency care in a range of countries.

thrombolytic treatment – 'door to needle time'. In primary care, keeping thrombolytic treatment available for the relatively rare occurrence of a heart attack in any one practice would be capital intensive and challenge supply arrangements. As a result of these considerations, the vast majority of thrombolytic treatment has, over the last 20 years, been given in hospitals and only relatively recently and in special circumstances, such as in the Grampian area where transfer to hospital takes a considerable time, has any co-ordinated attempt been made to provide thrombolytic treatment before transfer to hospital. This example illustrates how the changing of the design of the emergency care system is driven, not by the needs of patients, but by the power of the stakeholders in the system and the forces operating on it. Until the system is refocused on to the needs of patients and their families, issues such as bed blocking, trolley waits and red alerts (hospital closure) will remain immune to management interventions.

Dental care

The UK has equivocated as to whether it wishes to provide a comprehensive national dental service, free at the point of use in the same way it provides for medical service. As a result, private sector primary care dentistry has flourished at the expense of NHS primary care dentistry and the overall state of dental health in the UK compares unfavourably with that in Western Europe and the USA (*see* Figure 5.7). The forces determining change in the paradigm revolve around the economic power of individuals to buy private dentistry; the political will to fluoridate water supplies to prevent dental caries; and the financial incentives within both the NHS and the private sector to treat dental disease rather than promote oral health and prevent disease.

In the USA, personal funding has focused more on oral health and preventive dentistry, including orthodontics, and it would seem likely that in the UK as personal disposable income and wealth increases, so private sector dentistry will emphasise more orthodontic and preventive care.

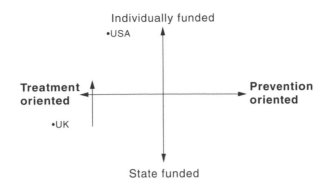

Figure 5.7: Orientation of dental care in the United Kingdom.

Systems

In Chapter 4 we considered primary care as a 'learning system' and the features that might contribute to enhancing it. Thinking of primary care as a system means seeing it as a whole, as discussed in this chapter's introduction. This means:

- looking at the inter-relationships between the elements of the system rather than at the elements themselves
- seeing the patterns of change within the system, how it is changing and evolving over time rather than taking static snapshots of the current situation
- looking at the 'physiology' of the system rather than its 'anatomy'.

The general principles involved in understanding how systems work have been developed from diverse fields such as social sciences, engineering and business management. Systems thinking also offers a set of specific tools and techniques for understanding how systems work.

- *Feedback* – where the consequences of an action feed back to influence the forces which led to that action. In biological systems, homeostasis is the feedback mechanism whereby the status quo is maintained. Temperature regulation, blood pressure and heart rate are, for example, all self-regulating, feedback, 'homeostatic' systems.
- *Servo-mechanisms* – derive from engineering. Consider for example servo-assisted brakes. The principle is that the efficiency of the system can be improved if the product of the action is used to amplify the forces producing the action. So, in a servo-assisted brake system, braking produces a vacuum, which amplifies the braking force. Consider how pupils dilate in poor light so as to maximise visual acuity or some of the ways adrenaline works to maximise the body's preparedness for stress as examples of servo-mechanisms in physiology.
- *Leverage* – in simple terms the use of levers enables the maximum change for the minimum effort. This means seeing where actions and changes in structures can lead to significant, enduring improvements in performance.

Leverage therefore follows the principle of economy of effort where major change is produced, not incrementally – dealing in health terms with the symptoms – but rather by understanding the pathology and disease process involved, so that we can treat the cause rather than the effect. It is hard to disagree with these principles but in most real life situations, it is not easy to see how to apply leverage.

Understanding, analysing and interpreting systems, seeing where the feedbacks, servo-mechanisms and leverage are operating or could be applied, will help us use and learn from our experience more effectively. In the primary care sector, we are so often focused on the day-to-day problems of patient demand, budget management and the process of balancing the demands made on us that we fail to see, analyse and understand the systems which are driving our performance. If we are to move away from symptomatic responses to appreciating the forces determining our actions, i.e. move from short-term 'band-aid' symptomatic treatment to a treatment of the underlying causes, then we need to use the principles and tools to start interpreting the systems. The purpose of systems archetypes is to help us to understand the systems, analyse the way they work and appreciate where leverage might be successfully applied to produce the maximum change for the minimum effort.

System archetypes
Supply-induced demand

The demand for healthcare will increase if more provision is made. The principle of supply-induced demand, which applies as much to soap powder as to coronary artery bypass grafting or surgery appointments, is that increasing the supply will stimulate demand, although this only applies in a system where there is unmet demand to be stimulated.

Box 5.2

Prestwood House Surgery, like all surgeries in the area, was experiencing pressure on the surgery appointment system. More patients seemed to want appointments than were available and, as a result, patients were waiting several days to see a doctor, some were attending casualty unnecessarily, some patients were making inappropriate 'just in case' appointments and some patients were not attending because they felt better before their appointment came up. More and more 'extras' were being fitted in at the end of surgeries and these consultations were often rushed and unsatisfactory. The temptation was to ask the doctors to provide more and more appointments to meet the demands of patients, but experience has shown that this has not worked in the past.

The experience of other surgeries has been that introducing a filter, through nurse or GP triage, may be a better, less symptom focused, approach. This means seeing the recurring theme or archetype of supply-induced demand and appreciating how leverage can be applied to change it. Leverage over access to primary care could come from skill substitution such as via nurse triage or from looking at the archetype differently. Supply-induced demand could look very different if 'expert patient' support groups or telephone triage arrangements are introduced. 'Technology changes ground rules' – or the archetypes operate differently in different circumstances.

Supply-induced demand is one of a small number of recurring patterns of structure or 'system archetypes' which between them form the key to understanding and interpreting any system. The system archetypes suggest that management problems are never unique, something that experienced managers know intuitively. If homeostasis, servo-mechanisms and leverage are the basic tools of system thinking, then system archetypes are analogous to the stories that get told again and again. Just as in the arts there are common themes which recur again and again in drama, art and literature, so also in the primary care sector a relatively small number of these archetypes are common and recur in a large variety of situations. The same archetypes occur in a variety of different sectors, e.g. economics, politics, science, business and healthcare, and it is this unifying approach which makes *system thinking* such a powerful tool.

Because archetypes are subtle, we may not recognise them when we first see them. Sometimes they produce a sense of *déjà vu*, but often it can be some time and only following a period of reflection before we realise what we are dealing with.

Mastering system archetypes sets an organisation on the path of putting system thinking into practice. It is not enough to say that we need to move from symptomatic, sticking plaster approaches to a more strategic and long-term planning approach – we need a way of doing it and systems thinking offers us a tool to help us with that transition. It is not even enough to see a particular structure underlying a particular problem – this can lead to solving that problem, but it will not change the behaviour, attitudes, beliefs and values that produced the problem in the first place. Only when such changes occur can we claim that the system is adapting to, or learning from, experience. For the primary care sector to become such a *learning system*, managers, clinicians and all those involved in the sector will need to change the way they look at things so that they can appreciate and learn from the forces that create their situation. The purpose of system archetypes is to recondition our perceptions, so as to be more able to 'see the wood and the trees' and to see where leverage can be usefully applied. Once a system archetype is identified, it will always suggest areas for change.

Although there are about a dozen different systems archetypes, they are all made up of the basic building blocks:

- reinforcing processes such as servo-mechanisms
- balancing process such as homeostasis
- leverage
- the effect of time.

We will now consider a number of other system archetypes from a primary care perspective and, although not exhaustive, this approach can help illustrate how understanding the systems, analysing, interpreting and gaining insight into the way they work, can help us improve the performance of the primary care sector.

Balancing process with delay

Description. When there is a delay between cause and effect, then appreciation of what is happening will lead to an exaggerated corrective action or failure to take any corrective action (*see* Figure 5.8).

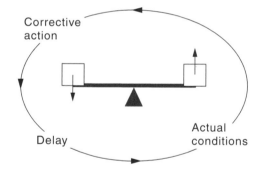

Figure 5.8:   Balancing process with delay.

Management principle. In a sluggish system where there is considerable delay between cause and effect, aggressive response can produce instability. The principle should therefore be: either be patient, or make the system more responsive by building in early warning systems, or feedback systems to stimulate the response, or restraining forces to dampen down exaggerated response.

Example. Consider the management of epidemics – particularly those involving time delays such as the human form of CJD or foot and mouth disease. In both cases, the fear of the effect of the infection on the individual and the community and the fact that there is a delay between awareness of the epidemic and the development of an understanding of the scale or numbers who are infected, leads to responses having to be made which may be either too muted or too exaggerated. The 'kill and burn' policy for foot and mouth and the removal of beef from school and restaurant menus in the CJD case, may seem like sensible ways of dealing with the problem but they are likely to end up as either over- or under-correction.

Limits to growth

Description. Success feeds on itself to produce a period of accelerating growth or expansion. Then the expansion slows because more and more energy is taken up maintaining the status quo rather than producing more success and growth. The growth phase for success is caused by reinforcing feedback processes. The slowing arises due to a balancing process, brought into play as a 'limit' approach. The limit can be a lack of resource or a response by internal or external stake-holders in the system to the growth.

Box 5.3:   An example

John took over a well-respected optician's business when David retired. David had been reducing his workload for some years, and initially, John was able to expand the business rapidly. His reputation spread and more and more people consulted him, so profits rose and he took on a second, then a third practitioner to help him. Soon, it became difficult to look after the number of customers wanting to consult – there were not enough rooms and the phone system, the secretaries and the parking spaces all became over-burdened. Then customers began to cancel their appointments – they couldn't park, the times were inconvenient or they had to wait too long to be seen. The response was 'I'd rather go elsewhere.' Growth in the business slowed dramatically, reputation suffered and enthusiasm waned.

Management principle. Don't push on the reinforcing growth process too hard. Instead deal with the processes and forces limiting growth, i.e. look out for parking places, phone systems and other infrastructure issues.

Shifting the burden

Description. A 'short-term solution' is used to correct the problem, with seem-ingly positive immediate results. As the same correction is used more and more, long-term, more fundamental options are used less and less and over time may be forgotten. In the end, fundamental or curative solutions are hardly considered at all.

Box 5.4:   Example – The prescribing budget

Drugs are expensive and the prescribing budget in primary care has been growing faster than inflation for many years. As a result, many practices are experiencing pressure on prescribing budgets and are being encouraged to reduce their costs. Short-term measures such as switching to generics, not prescribing drugs which can be bought over the counter, transferring costs into hospital budgets and stopping 'cosmetic' treatments will have some effect, but in the end the more fundamental solutions – such as encouraging patients' self-reliance and encouraging patients to stop smoking, to breast feed, to take more exercise and to lose weight – receive less and less attention as more and more focus is put on managing prescribing pressures.

Management principle. Focus on the fundamental solution. If symptomatic solutions are imperative because budget overspends have to be addressed, then use the short-term solutions to gain time while working on fundamental solutions (*see* Figure 5.9). Similar examples can be considered such as shifting the burden through using skill substitution or referring more to hospital while more fundamental solutions such as improving health, preventing disease and addressing the relationships between patient and provider might be more appropriate.

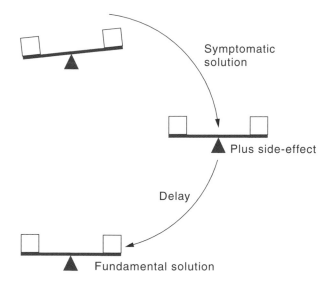

Figure 5.9:   Short-term and fundamental solutions.

Other examples of 'shifting the burden' where short-term 'quick fix' solutions seem to have a positive effect but store up long-term problems include the following initiatives.

- Waiting list initiatives which divert limited capacity or use the private sector.
- Expanding the number of appointment slots in surgeries to address increasing patient demand without considering other potential solutions to access difficulties, e.g. triage, group sessions, use of support groups and self-help programmes.
- Restricting the practice area or closing the 'list' as a way of coping with increase in population, e.g. a new housing estate, which simply 'shifts the burden' on to other neighbouring practices.
- Dealing with bed blocking by the elderly by seeking to make social services responsible and 'shifting the burden' into their budget rather than looking at the needs of the elderly across health and social care sectors and how these might be met.
- Introducing physiotherapy triage for orthopaedic problems prior to a consultant outpatient appointment. While this might sometimes be a more appropriate management plan for some patients, the use of it to reduce outpatient waiting times by simply introducing a two stop system may help short-term 'targets' without doing a great deal to improve the care that patients with orthopaedic problems receive.

The more you think about any aspect of healthcare, the more examples of 'shifting the burden' archetype will be found. It is perhaps fair to say that 'pass the parcel' would be an appropriate game for a health service Christmas party! In truth, this is not restricted to the health sector – shifting the burden between health and social care, between the health sector and the voluntary sector and between professional care and self-care are further examples. While it may well be appropriate to 'shift the burden' for the quality of care individuals receive, to improve the efficiency of the system and to target resources where they can most effectively be used, this is not always the case. The temptation has to be to transfer care and the cost of it from one sector or budget to another for short-term political or operational reasons without considering or giving due weight to the consequences.

Short-termism

Description. There is always the temptation, in any pressurised areas such as the primary care sector, to introduce short-term solutions at the expense of the long term. The vision of what we are trying to achieve can be constantly sacrificed to short-term performance standards, political demands or expediency. The delay involved in seeking long-term solutions always tends to reduce the weight that long-termism has in decision making. In particular, the annual financial and accounting processes of the NHS have promoted the focus on short-termism.

The idea that all the primary care practitioners in a local area would have an educational afternoon once a month so as to value education more highly, improve communications and thus the quality of care patients receive was the accepted vision of a group of 40 clinicians. However, this vision can easily be lost – or eroded – if short-term issues such as pressure on surgery appointments, difficulty in covering pharmacy shops and dental practice, etc. cannot be resolved. Fear of building up patient demand and making access to care more difficult, i.e. short-term pressures, can get in the way.

Other examples include the reviewing of repeat prescriptions, where the vision of reviewing a patient's medication at regular intervals with that patient can be repeatedly deferred because it is inconvenient.

Management principle. Hold the vision.

Escalation or competition

Description. Two individuals, teams or organisations see their security as depending on a relative advantage over the other. Whenever one gets ahead, the other is more threatened leading it to act more aggressively to re-establish its advantage, which threatens the first, increasing its aggressiveness, and so on. Often, each side sees its own aggressive behaviour as a defensive response to the other's aggression: but each side acting 'in defence' results in a build-up that goes far beyond either side's desires.[5] You only have to think of the volatile interaction between receptionist, doctor and demanding patient, when each side seeks to 'up the ante' and which can frequently spiral out of control, leading to aggressive behaviour and complaints, to realise how relevant this archetype can be. More broadly, independent contractor organisations competing with each other, e.g. pharmacists' shops, can end up with all parties being harmed rather than producing benefit.

As anyone who has investigated and arbitrated in complaint situations will realise, the way out is to look for 'win–win' areas for the parties. In many instances, the heat can be taken out of situations, over time, and the escalation spiral ended. This only happens when the parties realise that their behaviour is counter-productive.

Other examples include: (i) negotiating about outpatient appointments or waiting lists to try and gain 'competitive advantage' or earlier treatment; (ii) aggressive price cutting to gain market share in a retail outlet such as a pharmacy producing loss leaders; and (iii) the winding-up, manipulative, behaviour that so characterises the relationship between toddlers and their parents.

Management principle. Look for a way for all parties to win or achieve their objectives and try to persuade one or more parties to take 'peaceful' action to reduce the tension.

Success to the successful

Description. Support and resources rapidly transfer to individuals or organisations often at the expense of others. In any system or sector, this can lead to failure to keep the whole system in balance. While the football league with its promotion and demotion, crowds and competition may be a 'balanced system', there is no doubt that for Manchester United, Liverpool and Arsenal success breeds success.

In the healthcare sector, however, where it is important that all individuals and organisations provide high quality care, it is important to ensure that resources are allocated fairly on the basis of health need and do not flow inappropriately to the successful and powerful. Julian Tudor-Hart[7] points out that in the NHS the resources available for care are often inversely related to the needs of the population – areas of deprivation are often under-resourced compared to more affluent areas. This means that resources have flowed to those demanding health-care, e.g. rich affluent communities, at the expense of weak communities such as inner cities and deprived industrial areas.

Management principle. Look for the overarching goal that we are trying to achieve in the healthcare sector. In some cases, review the underlying mechanisms so as to ensure that the system remains balanced, so that elements in the system are not competing for the same limited resource. One of the fundamental reasons for the NHS being introduced was to produce a fairer system – success to the successful describes the tendency for this fairness always to be less than perfect.

Tragedy of the commons or diminishing returns

Description. A widely available service, such as a radiography department, is used by all clinicians on the basis of patient need. Initially, the service works well but eventually as more and more people use it, waiting times get longer and longer and the effectiveness of the service diminishes. Finally, the service can become next to useless, e.g. consider MRI scanning with an 18-month waiting list or an ultrasound service for the diagnosis of problems in early pregnancy with a 10 day waiting time. While short-term fixes to acute problems may be arranged, they can often simply shift the burden to other areas.

Management principle. The managing of the resource through educating every-one to use it efficiently, creating forms of self-regulation and peer pressure or agreed guidelines and access arrangements, helps to preserve the value of the resource and promote its usefulness.

Other examples in the primary care sector include '*go and see your GP*', which is used as an excuse for everything from certification to worries about health scares. The GP becomes a stress counsellor and waiting list manager to such an extent that the resource 'GP' is both difficult to access, over-burdened and unable to act as an effective primary care physician. Also consider the introduction of a counselling service into primary care, the development of new antibiotics and the emergence of antibiotic resistance.

Fixes that fail

Description. A short-term solution has unforeseen long-term consequences which need more and more treatment to fix them (*see* Figure 5.10).

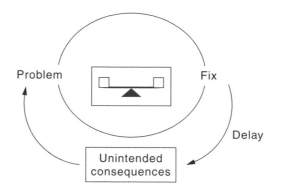

Figure 5.10:   Short-term fixes that fail.

Example. The use of antibiotics for post-operative wound infections where they have always worked in the past but as increasing resistance becomes a problem, more and more complex regimes are needed.

Other examples include: borrowing to pay interest on other loans or consolidating loans; cutting back on building maintenance or staff training to save costs – eventually leading to breakdowns and poor staff performance which again create more pressure for cost cutting in other areas.

Growth and underinvestment

Description. Growth approaches a limit, which can be eliminated or pushed into the future if the organisation or individual invests in additional capacity. But this investment must be aggressive and sufficiently rapid to prevent stalling or a reduction in growth, or else it will never be made. Frequently key goals or performance standards are lowered to justify underinvestment. When this happens, there is a self-fulfilling prophecy where lower goals lead to lower expectations, which are then borne out by poor performance caused by underinvestment.

Management principle. If there is a genuine potential for growth, build capacity in advance of demand, as a strategy for creating demand and managing it. Hold the vision, especially as regards assessing key performance standards and evaluating whether capacity to meet potential demand is adequate.

Example. The practice faces a rise in local population, producing increased demand and a rising list. The temptation is to meet this demand by incrementally increasing capacity but, in truth, provision has to be made to meet the needs of the practice when the development has been finished. Capacity has to be developed to deal with that end product rather than constantly increased by 'drip feeding'.

Other examples include the pressure on district nurses and maternity services caused by patients' earlier discharge from hospital without concurrent investment in the community. Another example is the growth in personal transport, such as cars, causing congestion due to government failure to invest adequately in the road network.

In whose interest?

Description. Things work the way they do because it is in the interest of the stakeholders that they work that way. Decisions to change the way things work, which challenge the interests of one or more stakeholders, particularly if they have power within the system, will be resisted and thwarted unless those stakeholders can be convinced that change is in their interest.

Example. The number of emergency admissions from primary care into hospital has been rising inexorably for many years. Tackling the rising number of emergency admissions has been seen as a way of preserving the capacity in secondary care to deal with elective admissions and promote the efficient use of resources, particularly accident and emergency and ambulance services. However, the increase in emergency admissions has been used by hospital trusts as a way of obtaining additional, non-recurrent resources to deal with the emergency admissions 'crisis' and, in addition, has been used by primary care practitioners to publicise the pressures they are under. In truth, 'shifting the burden' behaviour between primary and secondary care has been going on.

Another example within the primary care sector can be seen with prescribing. With more and more care provided in primary care, it is not surprising that the number of prescriptions and the costs of prescriptions have been rising faster than the rate of inflation. Nevertheless, it can be seen as 'in the interests' of the powerful stakeholders in the primary care sector to resist management initiatives which seek to maximise the efficiency and effectiveness of prescribing through the introduction of 'managed care' arrangements.

- The pharmaceutical industry is a major and powerful stakeholder in this system. It is in its interests to promote spending on drugs in primary care and the industry spends lavishly on marketing, supporting continuing professional development, 'joint ventures', audit and sponsorship. The profits made from drugs and the industry's interest in maintaining the current system, means that it is prepared to invest comparatively large amounts in promoting the interests of the existing system.

- GPs have been major prescribers of drugs (although following the Crown Report,[5] nurse and pharmacist prescribing is now developing) and wish to preserve their power and freedom to prescribe in their patients' interests, without interference from management, pharmacists and other non-GPs who 'don't understand' the importance of their clinical freedom, patient advocacy role and 'rights' to prescribe as they see fit.
- Patients, who see drug company marketing 'evidence' in the media, are often influenced by the attitudes and advice of friends, commercial pharmacies and primary care practitioners to increase their use of medication. It is not in their interests – as they are not direct funders – to question their need for drug therapy or to consider other approaches which may be more demanding of them in terms of change in behaviour, e.g. stopping smoking, losing weight, taking more exercise, receiving counselling or physiotherapy, etc.
- Health authorities, perversely, have not only found it difficult to tackle uncontrolled prescribing expenditure, but also have to reflect that it has been in their interest to have difficulty in this task. This difficulty has meant additional powers for them, the development of 'managed care' tools to tackle the autonomy and clinical freedom of primary care clinicians and drive the process of the development of corporate approaches in primary care including the concept of unified budgets where prescribing is seen as one option alongside other forms of care provision.
- Pharmacists make their profits from drug dispensing as well as other retail activities and it has been very much in their interests to work with the other stakeholders to expand drug spending.

As a result, 'failure' to tackle the marked variation in prescribing behaviour between practitioners and practices and the overspending on prescribing budgets which has so threatened other types of care and activity by PCTs and PCGs has been allowed to continue.

Other examples of 'in whose interest?' include the difficulty of establishing a 'National Institute for Primary Care' and the introduction of NHS Direct and walk-in centres; the antipathy of some GPs to the development of corporate organisations in primary care; the failure to tackle long waiting lists, which can sometimes be seen as in the interests of consultants wishing to fuel their private income; and the failure to increase the proportion of mothers who breast feed their babies, because it can be seen as in the interest of employers, baby milk manufacturers and hospitals to encourage bottle feeding.

Analogy

It's a bit like pushing a snowball uphill. It needs a lot of pushing if it's not to roll back and smother the pusher – but if everyone agrees it is worth doing, then it can be done!

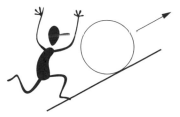

Management principle. Make sure change is seen as in the interest of the parties – especially those with power. Design the process of change towards an agreed vision with commitment and incentives.

Conclusion

Each of the above archetypes or recurring design themes illustrates how important the relationships between individuals and between issues, in appreciating how the system works, are. Between them they illustrate why understanding the 'balance' or relationship between the issues is important for those who manage, lead or seek to change the system. If they simply rely on understanding the anatomy of the primary care sector rather than the physiology of the primary care system, they will be like factory managers who know all about the widgets but nothing about the process of production and how it fits into the whole manufacturing system and the broader commercial sector. However, understanding the 'anatomy' really does matter because the 'physiology', the systems, the behaviour and the relationships can only be appreciated with a thorough grasp of such 'anatomical' knowledge.

- Appreciating the importance of leverage, incentives and disincentives in managing change.
- Understanding why individuals and teams may be reluctant to adapt and change.
- Understanding why so many aspects of care may fail to introduce evidence-based practice and remain stuck in a time warp.
- Understanding why some relationships in the primary care sector may be strong and persistent even though they can appear perverse and inappropriate from the outside.

- Appreciating why aspects of relationships such as frustration, dependency, supplicancy, and resentment can persist and even flourish despite the damaging effects that they can have on individuals.

The paradigms, models or patterns of the primary care sector provide another perspective on the performance of the sector. Rather than recurring themes, they are the way those themes are delivered or put together. The analogy of transport may be helpful – where the physiology of the internal combustion engine and the hydraulic braking system is delivered through private transport or public transport via the bus, the plane, the train and the car. Here, the archetypes are hydraulics and the internal combustion engine, and the paradigms are private transport, public transport and national airlines, which are each different approaches to delivering our need for increasingly flexible and efficient personal and group transport.

References

1 Senge PM (1993) *The Fifth Discipline. Business.* Random House Books, New York.
2 Starfield B (1994) Is primary care essential? *Lancet.* **344**: 1129–33.
3 Rivett G (1998) *From Cradle to Grave.* King's Fund, London.
4 Department of Health (2001) *National Service Framework: older people.* DoH, London.
5 Department of Health (1999) *Review of Prescribing, Supply and Administration of Medicines.* Crown Report. DoH, London.
6 Department of Health (1997) *The New NHS: modern, dependable.* DoH White Paper, London.
7 Tudor-Hart J (1988) *A New Kind of Doctor.* Merlin, London.

CHAPTER 6

The new paradigms

Introduction

The preceding chapters have analysed the heritage of the primary care sector and equipped us to judge how fit the sector is for its emerging responsibilities. There is, however, another aspect to making this judgement – we ought to consider where all this might be leading and whether current developments make sense in the light of such considerations.

The *Tomorrow's World* material, included on the website,[1] should now be read and listened to again so that readers can appreciate the rest of this section. This material was prepared as part of a scenario planning project run by Northwest Anglia Health Authority in the late 1990s and offers us two alternative views of how the primary care sector might look in a few years' time. Inevitably, neither of the described futures will be 'right' and each should, therefore, be regarded as cartoons or 'exaggerations to make a point'.

In this chapter, I shall consider how the current *paradigms*, considered in the previous chapter, can be expected to have evolved and adapted – if either of the two futures can be believed. This consideration will be supported by a critical analysis of the paradigms contained within the *futures* so that a more balanced judgement about the fitness of the sector can be attempted in the final chapters. An overview of the two alternative views of the future in *Tomorrow's World* is shown in Table 6.1, which summarises and compares some of the key aspects of the two pictures. It should be used to help clarify the text. This will provide us with a useful reference point when we compare how current paradigms might have adapted.

In the previous chapter we looked at the following paradigms.

- Whole service paradigms, with the NHS at the community funded end of the spectrum, compared to the United States which is at the self-funding end of the spectrum, with other countries falling in between. In addition we noted that the UK is moving from an institution, or hospital centred service, to a much more home centred service, in line with developments in other countries.
- Sector paradigms, where we looked at how the design of the primary care sector is evolving and changing in response to the forces acting on it.
- Professional paradigms such as the medical model. In these, we considered the extent to which the heritage of professional behaviour has equipped

Table 6.1:   Overview summary table of the provision of care in 2010

	Choice First	Feel Good Factor
Dynamics	• Unplanned • Market led • Quality assured	• Planned • Centrally regulated++
Welfare state	• Supervises personal investment accounts • Independent regulator	• Citizen/state contract • Pressure on poverty • Safety net
Philosophy	• Individual centred • Personal responsibility • More personal choice • Entrepreneurial • Closed decision making • Profits matter	• Public health • Personal responsibility • Less personal choice • Paternalistic • Open to scrutiny • Salaried service
Bio/social	• New genetics to protect profits • Liberated 'enfranchised' • Personal freedom	• New genetics as a planning tool • Incentives for conformance • Social engineering
Health promotion	• Peripheral – is it VFM? • Personal responsibility	• Core function • Corporate responsibility
Primary care	• Dominates+++ • Professionally directed • Accredited • Whither the GP?	• Dominates++ • Community directed • Regulated • Whither the GP?
Specialist care	• Centre for 3 000 000 • Specialist members of staff • 95% reduction in referrals	• Centre for 3 000 000 • Telelinks or dispatch • Referrals down 30%
Acute hospitals	• High tech partner • Outreach • ? Specialist members • Fewer and smaller	• Resource for community • Outreach • Fewer
Health/social care funding	• PIA • Insurance+ • Co-payment+++	• Welfare = H+S • Taxation+ • Co-payment+
Personal values	• Choice • Independence • Effectiveness • Autonomy	• Community spirit • Personal responsibility • Equity • Education
Medical science	• Interventionist • If it works • Research matters	• Prevention • Care matters • Your responsibility
Impact of technology	• Videophones • Iris security	• Electronic elections • Regulating teams

practitioners to work in teams and promote the autonomy of patients and service users at the same time as retaining their trust and respect. The extent to which professional behaviour is self-seeking, or driven by the interests of patients, might also considered.

We can now consider how each of these paradigms relates to the futures illustrated in Table 6.1. In doing so we will consider the range of influences operating on current paradigms and how they have contributed to the alternative futures.

Whole service paradigms

Whereas the NHS is centrally funded out of general taxation, free at the point of use and provided as a service to the whole community, the two alternative futures describe very different services.

The tensions inherent in the current NHS might be considered to stem from the following reasons.

- The extent to which the whole service is *centrally* directed or has its priorities more *locally* determined.
- The extent to which users of the service have *choice* and influence over the location, accessibility and quality of the service they experience as well as the freedom to change their service provider or get a second opinion.
- The extent to which individual *citizens' rights* have been given priority over their *responsibilities* and have challenged the power and *patronising paternalism* of care providers.
- The degree to which individuals trust the service when they feel that the *social contract* which has underpinned the service from the start – everyone invests when they are healthy so that they don't have to worry when they are sick – is less relevant in a modern society which seems troubled by immigration, more polarised between the majority of 'worried affluent fit' and the minority of 'disadvantaged scroungers', less altruistic, less tolerant and less trusting.
- The extent to which the government, as funder of the service, is prepared to meet the ever increasing cost of healthcare and the ever increasing proportion of the national income which is required to provide it. Recent announcements following the Wanless Report[2] indicate continuing acceptance of the communities' responsibility for the service – but this cannot be unlimited – even though the demand for resources seems insatiable. Interestingly, the question of limiting the NHS's responsibility to treating and preventing disease has been hardly considered. Excluding cosmetic services – nose jobs and hair transplantation – and lifestyle treatments – such as viagra and sports injuries – may seem easy but definitions are difficult in this area and as the population ages it is less tolerant of nature's variations and the ravages of time, so the tensions increase.

- How the service addresses its demonstrable problems such as inefficiencies, variation in quality and pockets of poor practice. These can sometimes only be safely addressed (it is assumed) by tighter central control, more performance management and tighter and tighter accountability frameworks, which inevitably reduce the ability of the service to be sensitive to the personal needs and preferences of individuals.

These tensions have led to very different arrangements in the two alternative futures (Table 6.1). In **Choice First** the power over resource allocation has been devolved to every individual. *Personal investment accounts* and a scheme of membership have served to balance the tensions between rights and responsibilities of individuals and of service providers. The result is that users and providers are much clearer about what they should expect and are entitled to in any given circumstance. In addition, there is a much stronger *quality assurance* ethic throughout the service and this has been reinforced by *competition* for members and a tendency for provider organisations to increase in size.

Whereas the NHS offered a fair system where everybody in the population had equal access to care, in Choice First, although there is a basic provision open to everybody, most people top up the basic care with additional voluntary contributions or co-payments and this has served to produce a disenfranchised minority of those who often have the greatest health needs and who often feel they have invested all their lives and have a right to be cared for.

It is interesting that although this is a professionally led and technically driven alternative, the vast majority of care is provided outside specialist centres, within the community. Technological developments have enabled devolution of care from hospital and the development of specialist centres serving much larger populations than traditional district general hospitals. This movement has served to promote personal responsibility and end the dependency culture which institutional care served to promote.

The **Feel Good Factor** on the other hand is a centrally funded system still based on the ethic of community responsibility. Capitation based funding does not provide everything so some top-up is permissible but is by no means essential. There is much more local control, within the community, over the policies to be followed and this has led to considerable restraint on personal freedoms, for instance, over diet, smoking, substance abuse, etc. Provision remains centrally regulated through Offhealth, ACE, etc., and the service is accountable to regional government for its use of resources and the quality of care provided. To some extent, this is a much more 'health of the public' focused service than the old NHS or Choice First so that priorities such as immunisation, disease prevention, health promotion, genetic responsibility and responsible personal behaviour are more valued. At the same time, it does have to deliver on strict central quality assurance requirements which cover not only the public health agenda, but also high quality specialist care when required. Specialist referral centres and rehabilitation centres have developed to serve larger populations, but referrals to them have decreased and several of the services they used to provide have been devolved into the community.

In both Choice First and the Feel Good Factor, the control of resources is through the primary care sector – individually controlled in Choice First and controlled via the community committee in the Feel Good Factor. The governing arrangements differ between the two futures. The directly elected committee in the Feel Good Factor is far more accountable to both users and funders than the traditional NHS. The call centre organisations in Choice First have to serve the needs of their members and shareholders, if they are to succeed in the competitive environment which Choice First describes.

Primary care sector paradigms

We noted in Chapter 4 that the 'primary care' paradigm in the United Kingdom has been evolving throughout the latter part of the twentieth century towards:

- a more team oriented provision of care with the individual citizen's relationship with the sector being less personal
- the governing arrangements of the sector becoming more corporate and more responsive to the needs of the community
- closer relationships between the constituent parts of the primary care sector, such as:
  - general medical practice
  - pharmacy
  - primary care nursing
  - social services
  - voluntary sector care
  - other professions working with primary care.

Best practice has dictated co-ordination and cohesion of care across traditional professional and organisational boundaries.

The Feel Good Factor

If we turn to the implications of the future described in the Feel Good Factor for the primary care paradigm, then there are a small number of themes to be considered.

Personal choice
This has been further restricted. Registration with the local Healthy Living Bureau is universal and while there may be some freedom to choose between different teams operated by the bureau, the locally elected committee and ethos

of community spirit implies a restriction on the individual's freedom to live any kind of deviant life. Social pressure to conform over a range of issues such as substance abuse, including smoking and alcohol; personal transport; exercise and health promoting behaviour such as breast feeding; supporting the handicapped and the elderly is encouraged.

Team focus

This future is driven by a team focus. The care and support provided by local teams is fundamental. Teams are judged on the effectiveness of the care they provide and the contributions individuals make to the team are valued, provided they contribute to effective team performance. Just as the Bureau is closely monitored by Offhealth and provides treatment in line with the advice issued by ACE, so local teams are judged by their performance against both these external standards and also by how their performance is perceived by the local community – as reflected by the elected committee.

We can anticipate that teams will seek to maximise their effectiveness by paying more emphasis to issues such as:

- *co-ordination of care* – where the skills and qualities of team members contribute to the overall package of care that is provided and where traditional professional boundaries are less relevant
- *clinical leadership* – we can anticipate that the personal responsibility of team members for the care they provide will be important to individual patients so that they know who is responsible and who to turn to if difficulties arise. The co-ordination of complex care packages will require clinical leadership. While it is clear that the process of leadership will be important, it would seem that this does not necessarily always have to be provided by the same individuals. We can envisage that the long-term support of a person with severe learning difficulties might be led by a team member with experience and training in the management or the care needs of such a handicapped individual; the care needs of a young single mother caring for a chronically sick child at home will need different skills. It is likely that each member of the team will lead on the management and support of a number of individuals and families. It may well be that administrative, ancillary and management skills to support the team will be centrally provided by the Bureau but that the era of *general management* where people without relevant clinical experience manage performance is over.

Co-ordination

The Bureau brings together all the various providers of primary care under one umbrella. Opticians, dentists, social workers, doctors, nurses, etc. all provide care for those registered with the Bureau – so the fragmentation, so apparent in earlier years in the NHS, has ended. The disjointed care of diabetics, for example, across optical services, chiropody, medical and nursing services, etc. has ended.

To meet the standards for the prevention of diabetic complications, it has [ ]
essential for care to be of the whole illness – its anatomy, physiology, biochemistry,
genetics, therapy, complications, sociology and psychology. To this can be added
the ethos that the Healthy Living Bureau is a broad *welfare* providing organisation
which sees its remit as extending well beyond physical and mental health and
into spiritual and community health.

Box 6.1: Case study – Julie's care in the Feel Good Factor

Julie is 39 and has had diabetes for 15 years. Both her parents developed it in
later life but she developed it in her first pregnancy. When she first developed
the condition she learned to inject her insulin and monitor her own glucose
levels. She attended the diabetic clinic at the hospital – 10 miles away – every
six months and, in addition, saw her optician and chiropodist annually, her
GP every four months, the practice nurse six-monthly and the diabetic liaison
nurse every few weeks. She went to the pharmacy for repeat prescriptions
every month, which involved an average of three phone calls and two trips
to the surgery. In all she calculated she lost 12 days' work each year just to keep
her diabetes properly monitored. Although everyone involved was helpful
and knowledgeable in their own field, they couldn't answer all her questions
and they rarely, if ever, all met together to discuss her clinical problems, her
concerns, her future and how to make her condition less of a burden.

Now, the Bureau co-ordinates her care. Twice a year she attends the
clinic and the eye, foot, diabetic, renal and psychology care workers see and
advise her. She has one of the new insulin implants, so no longer has to do
any injections and her levels are monitored by a telemetry link once or
twice a day. She knows there is a 30% chance that David (her son) will
develop diabetes but he has been fully immunised and is on the right diet
and exercise regime to keep this risk to a minimum. Jane and Louise (her
five-year-old identical twins) have no greater risk than the general population – the genetic worker at the Bureau did their SNIP profiles and what
a relief to her to have all this fully explained! Far from being frightened by
the genetics, it was a real relief and boost to her confidence to *know*.

Julie and Mike, her husband, have decided to try for another baby. The
Bureau has been supportive but only if they follow all the guidance. They
have advised them of the risks, arranged pre-conceptual testing to ensure
the baby is not at risk, and arranged specialist pregnancy care at the referral
centre, with increased telemetry monitoring and placental function care.
Julie knows she must not smoke, drink alcohol or take any medication
without it being recommended by her medicines manager – she knows
what to eat, how to keep herself fit and who to contact when she conceives.
Mike knows how to look after Julie, how to minimise the chance of his
sperm causing any difficulties and the role he will be expected to play in
pregnancy and family life.

Funding

The Bureau receives its funding from central allocation as a result of national policy over taxation, etc. Some additional top-up insurance is available but the activities of the Bureau are seen as a community responsibility and the social contract which has underpinned the health service from the start survives.

Choice First

Compared to the NHS in the latter part of the twentieth century, this future represents a radical change for the primary care paradigm. The themes which have dominated the development path of First Call simply reflect the dominant social themes of the early part of the new millennium. All important are quality assurance, alongside the rapid development of information technology and the requirement for providers of healthcare to demonstrate cost and clinical effectiveness, and efficient use of resources, alongside ease of access and a responsiveness to the views and requirements of every citizen.

Governing arrangements

Call centres such as First Call are increasingly large private sector organisations, raising capital from shareholders and the market. Some of the organisations, such as First Call, are run as 'not for profit' organisations, but increasingly there are pressures to commercialise. The capital intensive nature of delivering services in this high tech future requires a capital base and an investment programme, which only the market can generate. The organisation encourages both its staff and members to become shareholders so as to promote a sense of personal responsibility. This is also encouraged by the government contributing funds via personal investment accounts, rather than directly funding the organisation. Personal investment accounts encourage individuals to take more personal responsibility for their own health and also encourage personal contributions to the promotion of health and the running of the organisation.

First Call is run by a board of directors, just as any other private sector company, and it is they who are responsible for the organisation's performance and are accountable to the main funder – the government – for the organisation's performance, both in financial and clinical quality terms.

Beyond the basic funding provided through the personal investment account, additional resources are accessed by health insurance schemes and personal contributions. This has served the affluent community well but has led to a disenfranchised minority whose needs are inadequately addressed.

Personal choice

Control over one's own personal investment account and the fact that the need for face-to-face consultation has decreased, means that the individual service user has more real personal choice over their primary care provider. Although there are fewer organisations and they are each much larger, the use of information technology such as call centres, video consulting, etc. has encouraged choice and responsiveness to users' views. There is, however, some concern that the rapid consolidation of the primary care provider sector is reducing choice – as in the banking sector – and that government may have to step in to prevent further consolidation 'in the public interest'. Although personal choice over your care provider is important, so too is choice over what care is provided. In Choice First you get what works, but not necessarily what makes you feel special, comfortable, happy or simply better. These may only be available if you pay extra.

Box 6.2:   Case study – Julie's care in Choice First

Julie is 39 and has had diabetes for 15 years. Both her parents developed it in later life but she developed it in her first pregnancy. When she first developed the condition she learned to inject her insulin and monitor her own glucose levels. She attended the diabetic clinic at the hospital – 10 miles away – every six months and, in addition, saw her optician and chiropodist annually, her GP every four months, the practice nurse six-monthly and the diabetic liaison nurse every few weeks. She went to the pharmacy for repeat prescriptions every month, which involved an average of three phone calls and two trips to the surgery. In all she calculated she lost 12 days' work each year just to keep her diabetes properly monitored. Although everyone involved was helpful and knowledgeable in their own field, they couldn't answer all her questions and they rarely, if ever, all met together to discuss her clinical problems, her concerns, her future and how to make her condition less of a burden.

Since she has become a member of First Call she feels much more in control of her life – she manages her personal investment account alongside her bank account and supplements it by voluntary work with the diabetic group and by a regular savings plan to buy additional cover for possible diabetic complications. First Call co-ordinates her care – she sees the diabetic team twice a year and paid a supplement to get one of the new implantable insulin pumps as soon as they were developed. Recently the team have told her of new evidence that cardiac, neural and renal complications can be avoided by a cocktail of dietary supplements, drug treatments costing 100 euros per month and retroviral immunisations. If the RCT comes out showing more than 10% reduction in complications then Julie has decided to go for it. First Call will support her, paying 20% of the costs and she thinks it's a good deal. She knows there is a 30% chance that David (her son) will develop diabetes but she has done everything to keep his risk to a minimum. Jane and Louise (her five-year-old identical twins) have no greater risk than the general population – the genetic specialist at First Call did all their SNIP profiles and it was great to know the exact position so she and Mike (her husband) could plan ahead.

Julie and Mike have decided to try for another baby. They know the risks, have both been tested to make sure their sperm and ovaries are up for it and are going to use PCT (pre-conceptual genetic screening) to ensure the baby's risk of diabetes is minimised. They plan to pay the gold pregnancy supplementary insurance so Julie can be off work through most of the pregnancy. Mike and a carer can help for a few weeks after the birth and Julie will be covered for any complications.

Provision of care

This future represents a marked evolution from the *professional* based care of previous years. Radical change to the training programmes and the career structure have affected doctors, nurses, pharmacists, opticians, chiropodists, physiotherapists, etc. and this has followed and built on the experience of skill substitution and role development, such as went on with the development of nurse practitioners, nurse prescribing and nurse triage. There is a basic generic training followed by a period of working towards additional qualifications. This gives the organisation considerable flexibility in its clinical workforce but some staff found the changeover quite traumatic.

Co-ordination of care

The vast majority of care is now provided in the community via First Call and it is this organisation which co-ordinates the care people receive. The extensive use of information technology to record all clinical encounters and maintain a comprehensive clinical record which is accessible to all care providers in the organisation, means that care is much more co-ordinated than in the past. The fact that so few cases have to be referred on to referral centres and that much specialist treatment is also provided through First Call has meant much better co-ordination between specialist and generalist, than was the case between general practice and district general hospitals.

Key themes

It is clear from these two descriptions of the sector paradigms that two elements in particular differ fundamentally in the two futures.

1   The distinction between *personal* and *community* responsibility. While in Choice First personal responsibility is encouraged through personal investment accounts, membership status and the promotion of a choice ethic, in the Feel Good Factor personal freedom is restricted in favour of community spirit and although individuals are strongly encouraged to behave responsibly, it is peer pressure from the community rather than financial incentives which is the instrument to apply leverage.

2   The route by which the primary care organisation is *resourced* and then uses the resource to manage the delivery of healthcare through the NHS is different. In Choice First core funding is provided by government funding of personal investment accounts but considerable top-up funding is required and this promotes personal choice and responsibility. In the Feel Good Factor universal registration attracts the vast majority of the resources necessary for the provision of the Healthy Living Bureau's welfare services. Individuals are free to buy additional services but this is regarded as supplementary or luxury funding rather than any contribution to core services.

At the heart of these distinctions is the view taken about the role of the individual citizen and the community in being responsible for maintaining and improving health. Throughout the history of the NHS, there has had to be a balance struck between: (i) the universal right of every citizen to free healthcare, funded centrally through taxation, and the incentive for each citizen to take responsibility for maintaining his or her own health; and (ii) the citizen's responsibility to maintain his or her own personal physical, mental, spiritual and emotional health and promote health in others by behaving as an active, mature and enfranchised member of the local community and broader society.

In Choice First the balance has been tilted towards the promotion of 'empowered citizenship', while in the Feel Good Factor the balance has been tilted towards the strength of the local community. While neither of the descriptions is likely to be a blueprint for how the NHS will develop, this analysis does help to illustrate some of these key themes which health service practitioners and planners will need to consider as new primary care organisations develop.

Other key elements and issues which will need to be considered can be illustrated by considering the professional paradigms and service paradigms and how they differ in the Feel Good Factor and Choice First. The use of diagrams such as that shown in Figure 6.1 can be useful to help separate out the characteristics which distinguish what the alternative future is. These key themes form the axis of the diagram and combinations of them were used by the participants in the *Tomorrow's World* workshops (see the website for list of participants). It was at these workshops and in the discussions around them where the use of scenario planning techniques (see the IDON[3] website) led to the development of the two alternative futures which this section is based on.

Professional paradigms

In Chapter 5 we considered several aspects of the medical model and how they had contributed to the professional paradigm as a characteristic of the first half century of the NHS (*see* also Figure 6.1). Professions are characterised by:

- a common body of knowledge which members acquire through training and education and maintain throughout their professional lives

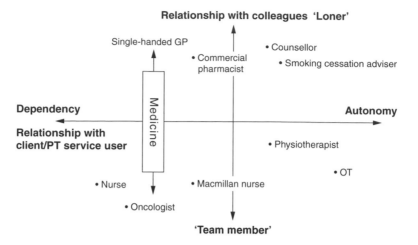

Figure 6.1:   Professional paradigms.

- maintenance of a register of professional practitioners which ensures professionals are qualified to practise
- adherence to a code of 'Standards of Practice' or an ethical framework underpinning the attitude of the professional to their practice.

While we can see from Figure 6.1 that the extent to which different professions in the primary healthcare sector view their relationship to each other:

- as team players
- as independent practitioners relating through referral or formal delegation

and the relationship with those consulting them as:

- promoting patient autonomy

or

- carers in a relationship of dependency, where the professional maintains control,

these are matters of degree rather than absolute.

The outcomes are the result of:

- the rapid expansion of the knowledge required to practise as a professional in healthcare delivery
- new developments in technology, such as open access to information via television and the Internet.

So, the role of the professional practitioner as the 'font of all wisdom' has changed. Access to the Internet, universal education and, in particular, development of higher education along with the plethora of healthcare programmes on television and radio have all served to demystify healthcare and challenge this aspect of professional behaviour. Increasingly, professionals are interpreting situations, symptoms and information, supporting individuals in times of adversity and adapting their advice depending on the individual circumstance they are dealing with. They are recommending treatment rather than insisting – 'doctor's orders', 'take your medicine', or 'nurse knows best' are becoming historic relics. In addition, as the service moves from being focused on the management of disease towards being focused on the maintenance and improvement of health, the move is more towards promoting autonomy, and away from the dependency relationship which characterised the design of the service and professional behaviour in past years. In addition, the trend has been away from individual professionals acting in isolation and towards them collaborating and working more closely together as members of a healthcare team, where they contribute their own professional expertise to common goals. In Choice First, we can see how access to information and support through the use of information technology, such as NHS Direct, has changed many aspects of the professional paradigms. Skill mix and skill substitution have led to radically different ideas about the role of healthcare specialists, general practitioners, nurses, pharmacists, etc.

'Grandfather' arrangements may allow GPs and others to continue to offer their experience and expertise at a time when the new accreditation system and training programmes are integrating all the healthcare professions within a common culture and ethical framework. But these arrangements are transitional and will end as the practitioners involved retire or leave.

Each practitioner is focused on ensuring First Call meets strict quality targets and on providing an effective and efficient system. In addition, each is focused on continuing personal development, succession planning and ensuring that all treatments are based on best evidence. The ethic of 'personal care' is less dominant than it was in the early years of the NHS.

Nursing has moved a long way from its charitable and care providing roots in Victorian times or even before. As a result of the social revolution of the twentieth century and the rise of professionalism, nursing has adopted aspects of the medical body of knowledge, covering nurse prescribing, nurse practitioner roles, specialist nursing practice and nurse triage. Each of these has helped to provide a more fulfilling career for nurses and preserved the relatively limited and scarce resources of the medical profession for the management of pathology. Caring for individual patients in times of need – bed bathing, comforting and providing personal care – has become less of a key nursing role and more a role for healthcare assistants and family members. While some specialist nursing groups such as Marie Curie and Macmillan nurses continue to see their primary role as providing personal care, others such as specialist outreach dialysis, diabetes, asthma and cardiac rehabilitation specialists have a much more specialist and advisory role.

In the Feel Good Factor, the extent to which professionalism dominates the policies and practice of the Healthy Living Bureau is much reduced. The electronically elected committee sets the policies and determines the pathway to achieving the tough targets sets by ACE and the government. This is a much more health centred service as opposed to a disease management service and, as such, the power of the professions as 'holders of the flame' has declined. All care providers have the same basic training up to NVQ level 4 although 'grandfather' arrangements have provided continuity for previous professional groups such as pharmacists and GPs. Even they have been expected to change their roles to a much more generic care provider role and health-promoting role. Many have resisted these changes and found the transition in mid-career difficult. However, the job security provided by the Bureau and the opportunities for further personal development have been attractive and persuaded most people to change rather than leave their profession.

Care is provided by healthcare teams – core people with common skills – and there are a number of specialists, some of whom provide care for several teams. Personal development workers help people facing change in their own lives such as retirement, family development or relocation. The teams are supported by extensive use of information systems, which monitor their performance as a team, as well as provide the team with the information and data necessary to support their role. The team is set performance goals, has responsibility as a team and is monitored as a team. They regularly meet to discuss the care plans for people requiring active intervention and they are expected to support each other and cover for each other's skill gaps and absences. Team members monitor each other, appraise each other and train each other as part of promoting team cohesion.

Community and holistic services covering healthcare, social care, etc. maintain a strong paternalistic and caring ethos. Although voluntary contributions and efforts are encouraged and rewarded, the role of individual team members in providing personal care and development remains strong.

In considering the implications for the current professional paradigms of the two alternative futures, it is clear that both of them represent a considerable challenge to the current paradigm. That paradigm, which has evolved over generations to suit the circumstance of the time and the circumstance of the relationship between care seeker and care provider, is seen as needing to adapt to new circumstance. The new circumstance encompasses:

- a service which is focused on promoting the health of the population rather than focusing on individual disease
- a service which is focused on a broader definition of health encompassing emotional, spiritual, physical and social health
- a service which is driven by the needs of the local community or its membership rather than the views of the care providers or imposed national policy.

The national role is seen as quality assurance and regulation rather than the detailed management of performance
- the devolution of power to the citizen, either acting individually as a 'member' or through an elected committee. This is seen as a counterweight to the power of vested interest groups such as professions and particular patient interest groups and as a promoter of a sense of personal responsibility for personal and individual health as well as being a broader constituent of social responsibility.

Box 6.3:   Case study – Nigel and Carol

Nigel has been a GP for over 20 years. He was senior partner, a PCG board member and a GP trainer. Carol, his wife, trained as a nurse but then had 10 years as a housewife and mother before returning part time as a bank nurse in the community.

- Since the Bureau arrived under the banner of the Feel Good Factor, Nigel has been grieving – he seriously considered early retirement but couldn't afford it. The surgery has been sold to the Bureau, all the staff have new jobs – most are doing additional training, but he is too old for all that. He still enjoys seeing patients but has to admit he is delighted to be freed from some of the trash he used to deal with and is beginning to enjoy advising on genetic therapy, using the new scanner and teaching. Carol thinks the Bureau is the best thing since sliced bread. She is an elected committee member and has become a specialist adviser to the family centre – coping with bedwetting, teenage tantrums and family discord. She still drives her old Morris Minor to visit the elderly at home – dressings and tea, tests and chat – but so many more are now cared for by their families: what a transformation.
- Nigel is now a director of Choice First – he is worried by the financial burden and thinks they should sell out to the bank. As a specialist practitioner he has dusted the mothballs out of his white coat, retrained to cope with all the new technologies and thinks the next 10 years – before retirement – are a really exciting opportunity. Carol has retrained too. As a videophone operator and adviser she works 18 hours a week – often in the evenings so the children and care for the old folks at home are not affected. She worries about having to pay for so much care for her mother and is skimping on her own insurance as a result. The children are now grown up and pretty independent but only because she and Nigel invested most of their savings and inheritance in care bonds so the children could start families with a clean slate.

Particular care paradigms

In Chapter 5 we looked at two of the sector paradigms as they have developed during the first half century of the NHS but mentioned that there were several other paradigms, which could warrant similar analysis. In looking at emergency care and dental care, we focused on the pattern and location of provision and the extent to which the paradigms were focused on disease or health. In this section, we will look at two of the other care paradigms and how each is dealt with in the two alternative futures – Choice First and the Feel Good Factor. In choosing to look at *elective care* and *rehabilitation*, it should be clear that this is done in order to illustrate how and why the paradigms have changed rather than to imply that many of the other paradigms including emergency care and dental care will have been unaffected. The description of the two futures should enable us to deduce implications for other sectors and areas of care and it is the use of these descriptions to deduce implications and compare alternatives which makes the use of 'scenarios' an exceptional planning tool.

Elective care
Feel Good Factor

Most elective care is now provided by the Bureau teams with the help of attached 'specialists' from the Phys rehab centres. Anyone needing inpatient care will be admitted to the regional research and referral centre, which serves a population of about three million people. This marks a radical change in the provision of elective care compared to the first half century of the NHS where district general hospitals provided the majority of elective care and served populations, sometimes less than 300 000. The change in the funding streams, so that PCGs and PCTs became responsible for the vast majority of NHS resources in the late 1990s, has led, in this model, to a devolution of specialist elective care into the community and home and to a consolidation of specialist, hospital based care to serve larger populations. Technological change has meant that elective surgery for hernias, cataracts and cholecystectomies, etc. no longer requires hospital admission, while new drugs, early interventions and preventive strategies have reduced the need for elective referrals by a third compared to the current situation where referrals are continuing to rise.

Figure 6.2 illustrates the fundamental change introduced as a result of *The New NHS: modern, dependable*[4] in 1997. Giving primary care control over resource allocation, so that hospitals are seen as a subcontractor of primary care has led, in this model, to an accelerated transfer of care from hospitals to the home because resources have also been transferred. The problem, throughout the late

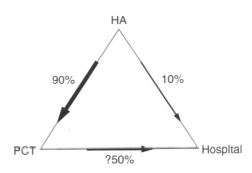

Figure 6.2: Fundamental change introduced as a result of *The New NHS: modern, dependable* in 1997.

twentieth century, of care being transferred from hospital without resources, with consequent stresses and strains on primary and community care, has been overcome. The consequences of such transfer of care without resources included:

- blaming primary care for overspending, e.g. GP drug budgets
- blaming primary care for rising emergency admissions as a result of treating patients with 'increasing dependency' at home
- difficulty over access to primary care services because of capacity and skill shortages
- resentment at the practice of shifting responsibility from cash limited budgets in the hospital sector into non-cash limited budgets in primary care without transferring the money. Because of the design of the primary care sector where independent contractors live off their bottom line of these non-cash limited budgets, the result was pressure on independent contractors' take home pay. In this future, the way that resources flow through primary care has been used to drive investment, skills substitution and devolution of specialist care and, allied with technological development and the resurgence of community spirit, has produced a much healthier, less healthcare dependent situation.

Choice First

Choice First has similarly seen changes in the way elective care is provided. Technological advance has seen a range of treatments, previously provided in hospital, now provided via local treatment clinics without admission to specialist referral centres. Table 6.2 gives examples.

The clinic has the latest diagnostic technology and most treatment plans in the home which result will be monitored by call centre staff. The need for additional specialist services has been reduced and district hospitals with their 'serried ranks for beds' have been relegated to the history books. Long-term care

Table 6.2:   Hospital treatments of the past we now usually find in history books

What we used to do	What we do now
Surgical removal of tonsils	If necessary, freeze and apply medical absorption
Coronary artery bypass surgery	Medical prevention of heart disease
	Arterial damage; laser surgery only if necessary as last resort
Surgical hernia repair	Medical/laser treatment for hernia
Endoscopy	Laser treatment
Arthroplasty – joint replacement	Regrowth of damaged cells and joint ligaments
Surgical prostatectomy	Drug treatment to reduce enlarged glands
Hysterectomy	Endometrial ablation and drug treatment
Cataract removal surgery	Use external applications to melt cataracts; laser/micro-surgery if required to correct vision

is no longer the responsibility of First Call and is dealt with by personal insurance plans. The development of nurse practitioners, the devolution of specialist medical care from hospital into the community and the developments of modern information technology, especially video and telemetry, has meant that compared with 1999 we refer less than one in twenty of the members we would have previously done. Bed usage is now less than 10% of 10 years ago and attitudes have changed so that members expect to be seen and treated by First Call and at the treatment centre, rather than attending or being admitted to hospital.

Technology has driven change in practice, change in professional roles and, most profoundly, change in attitudes from members as a result of personal investment accounts which have served to produce a future where elective care is provided, without waiting lists, when it is needed by individual members.

The use of private hospitals by the NHS to provide extra capacity, the development of new specialist referral centres, concentrating on elective surgery and the upgrading of community hospitals as local 'walk-in' and 'treatment' centres, can all be seen as experiments by the PCT led NHS in the early years of the new century, to adapt towards the kind of future described in Choice First.

Rehabilitation

For the first half century of the NHS, there has been little incentive for the primary care sector to invest time, energy and resources into rehabilitation. Recovery and convalescence are considered as normal physiological responses to illness or interventions such as surgery and, apart from emotional support, certification, any necessary nursing care and, where appropriate, the support of physiotherapy and occupational therapy, nature has been allowed to take its course. In secondary care, rehabilitation medicine, often allied to rheumatology, has developed as a specialist area supporting those with chronic disease and helping them adapt their lifestyles to cope with their chronic condition. Rehabilitation for individuals suffering acute illness, such as cardiac disease, has also developed as a specialist service to try and prevent recurrence, reduce dependency on the NHS and promote return to a happy and healthier state.

Choice First focuses primarily on personal responsibility and choice. In this model, the health service no longer pays for long-term care and support – individuals are expected to take out health insurance to meet these needs. As a result, we can anticipate that individual members of organisations such as First Call will be very keen to recover from acute illness and remain independent when they have chronic illness, so that they do not fall outside the net of care provided by First Call. Agreed treatment programmes are likely to include recovery and rehabilitation, even if some elements of this require insurance or personal contribution as a top-up. The story of Vikram, after he broke his legs skiing, illustrates this approach[1] but then he has a choice:

- patients who suffer a disabling event in their lives, such as a stroke or traumatic amputation
- patients born with an inherited or congenital health problem
- patients who develop disabling chronic conditions such as lung or connective tissue disease

will all find that their membership of First Call does not meet all their health needs. Their needs for rehabilitation, for long-term care, along with their physical and emotional needs to promote their independence and autonomy, will be met through insurance or their own personal funding or that of their family. The loss of income involved and the loss of choice that they will experience may make them worse off than they are in the current health service. It is worth reflecting that the bed blocking problem – which has caused so many 'knock on' difficulties with waiting lists and emergency admissions in the 1990s – has only been resolved in this future by restricting funded care and transferring responsibility into individual patients' hands.

In contrast, the predominant community spirit ethos of the Feel Good Factor with its broad care and welfare approach means a more supportive environment for anyone with rehabilitation requirements. Programmes of care agreed between the Bureau and individual citizens may limit individual freedom and choice but should offer those with ongoing care needs appropriate supportive packages. In this model, we can anticipate an increase in the rate of investment in services supporting physical recovery (such as physiotherapy) and those which promote independence (such as occupational therapy) to help individuals maximise their personal contribution to the community.

These two models offer a very different approach to rehabilitation. First Call is essentially a high quality acute intervention service, designed to meet the needs of the young and fit and the affluent majority with top-up health insurance. The Healthy Living Bureau is a public health oriented service, looking to promote the health of the community including coping with its inherent burden of disease. These alternative models differ fundamentally on whether they accept long-term health problems, be they inherited or acquired as a personal or community responsibility. As illustrated above, the Feel Good Factor and the current NHS share similar approaches to rehabilitation services with responsibility lying with the community and the individual citizen lacking any real power to change provision. Inevitably, the very different approach seen in Choice First challenges us to consider the place of 'personal power' and 'personal responsibility' but also to consider the risks of this approach to the health status of those with rehabilitation and continuing care needs.

References

1 www.radcliffe-oxford.com/challenge
2 Wanless D (2002) *Securing Our Future Health: taking the long-term view.* HM Treasury, London. www.hm-treasury.gov.uk/wanless
3 IDON (1997) IDON Scenario Thinking. IDON Ltd. www.idongroup.com
4 Department of Health (1997) *The New NHS: modern, dependable.* DoH White Paper, London.

CHAPTER 7

New responsibilities

Introduction

Chapter 6 used the material from the two *Tomorrow's World* scenarios (see www.radcliffe-oxford.com/challenge) to examine how the paradigms or models involved in primary care were evolving, and how they might continue to evolve over the next few years. This chapter looks at the responsibilities of current primary care organisations, how they are designed to discharge these responsibilities and how they might evolve with their responsibilities. We shall again use the material contained in the *Tomorrow's World* scenarios, Choice First and the Feel Good Factor, as reference points, but will not be constrained by these two alternatives in considering some of the issues that current primary care organisations are grappling with and those which are emerging as time passes.

Until recent times, the primary care sector in the United Kingdom has had two main responsibilities as:

- a *provider* of healthcare
- and as a *gatekeeper* to specialist care.

In addition, the sector has had a range of other important responsibilities including:

- sickness certification – validating healthcare status for third parties such as employers, benefits agencies and insurance companies
- continuity of care – including maintaining the lifetime health record and co-ordinating care across the primary care team and between home and hospital.
- liaising with other welfare agencies, such as the voluntary sector, social services, housing and the DVLA, acting as the patient's agent.

Although each of these remains important for the sector to discharge, they no longer represent its full spectrum of responsibilities. As discussed elsewhere in this book, the responsibilities of the primary care sector are evolving as a result of the forces acting on it. The new responsibilities considered in this chapter are partly an evolution of previous ones and partly transfers from other members of the health and welfare family.

Transfer of responsibilities to the primary care sector has been constrained until recent times for the following reasons.

- *Lack of accountability* of independent contractors in the primary care sector for their use, allocation and transfer of resources. Health authorities have commissioned secondary care and been able to hold that sector to account for the quality of its financial and clinical performance in a way they have been unable to match in primary care. Public health departments have been focused on supporting such commissioning work and delivering change in clinical practice in the light of emerging evidence and have been heavily involved in supporting the development of commissioning by health authorities. In the primary care sector, the inflexibility of national contracts, such as the *Red Book* or pharmacy regulations, has meant that primary care has largely operated outside the NHS performance management framework and outside the commissioning network of NHS trusts, public health and health authorities. As a result, primary care has not been held directly to account for the quality of its financial and clinical performance.

Primary care providers have also suffered as a result of the lack of accountability between them and health authorities and specialist NHS trusts. The transfer of work and responsibilities from secondary care, without adequate resources, has increased the workload and responsibilities of primary care providers over recent years and sometimes reduced their profitability – or at least required them to invest more capital in their businesses, for limited return.

Shortening length of stay in hospital because new technology permits earlier discharge, the emergence of private provision for the elderly, those with learning disabilities and those suffering from mental health problems, the therapeutics revolution, and the application of new technologies such as telecommunications, near patient testing and microprocessors outside hospitals have all contributed to this devolution of care and have all served to highlight the lack of accountability and the risks that poses to all parties.

- *Lack of trust.* Open book arrangements, regular performance reviews, secondment and shared posts, career paths with experience across agencies and sectors, joint finance and joint projects have all helped to build trust between health authorities, NHS trusts and social service departments. Primary care has been largely excluded from these arrangements and the trust enhancing relationships which emerge. As a result primary care organisations and those working in them frequently mistrust other sectors of care and the feeling is, too often, mutual. Trust is required between all the parties involved, if care is to be safe, if investment is to be safe and if careers are to be safe. If health authorities and hospitals don't trust primary care and primary care providers mistrust them, then transferring responsibilities, resources, etc. into primary care is just not safe and won't happen. Only when the parties trust each other and the system, will the potential benefits of high quality care outside hospital be realised. In the meantime, the lack of trust has been deeply damaging.

- *Continuity.* The relationships involved in the provision of primary care services often continue over many years in an intermittent and frequently unmanaged fashion.[1] Long-term relationships characterise the sector, independent contractors' investment in their business is long term, making career flexibility and mobility problematic. The transitory nature of health authorities and their staff, rapid change in NHS trust management and social service department staff, have tended to exaggerate the isolationist tendencies of primary care. Because there is less of a culture of long-term continuity and perceived unreliability in these other sectors, primary care – and especially GPs – sometimes feel it is they who are left holding the baby when everyone else moves on. This fear of being unsupported and of being left exposed to pick up the pieces constrains primary care providers from enthusiastically grabbing new responsibilities. General practitioners have always felt they have been the wicket keepers of the NHS team – expected to pick up all the pieces, catch everything and answer everyone's questions. People the system can't cope with, such as those with personality or behaviour problems, are discharged back to the GP; if there is a health scare people are told to ask their GP; care after five on a Friday, over bank holidays or in the middle of the night all seem to head the GPs way – without the kind of organised, systematic back-up which would make them feel safe. This feeling of continuing, unsupported responsibility also affects other independent contractors such as pharmacists and dentists, staff such as district nurses and health visitors and the broader groups such as the voluntary sector workers and carers.

Attempts to change the way the primary care sector has related to the rest of the NHS, such as the GP fundholding scheme, locality commissioning and total purchasing during the 1990s, can be seen as experiments to test whether enfranchising primary care can make specialist services more responsive to the healthcare needs of the community.[1] As the forces unleashed by the social revolution and technological revolutions have increased the potential power and responsibilities of the primary care sector, so the requirement for trustworthiness, accountability and the development of the performance management framework within which primary care's power and responsibilities can be balanced, have emerged. The Audit Commission's report into GP fundholding[2] showed some limited development of a more corporate approach to the provision of care, but without any convincing evidence of health improvement as a result. While fundholding, etc., added a new dynamic into the NHS system and served to illustrate that there are viable alternatives to the monolithic, bureaucratic, centrally driven NHS, there was little evidence that it was effectively tackling:

1   *The inverse care law*[3] whereby the NHS has often provided best care and most resources where the needs are limited, and the least well endowed care where the healthcare needs are greatest. Micro-resourcing through fundholding without any process (analogous to the Resource Allocation Working Party (RAWP)) to transfer resources from affluent areas to the most deprived, along with the process of deriving and developing fundholding budgets based

on historic utilisation patterns rather than on any analysis of healthcare needs of the local population, did not help.

2   *Health versus disease.* The fundholding unit was the GP practice whose history and culture was the management of disease. Health promotion clinics, screening, disease prevention and self-care were responsibilities which were 'bolted on' to general practice without adequate resourcing and which fundholding practices failed to fully absorb, develop and adapt to.

3   Too many practices in the fundholding schemes saw their responsibility as to their own patients, rather than to the whole community. Maverick practices negotiating special deals on behalf of their patients often bred resentment across the rest of the NHS family and, while often appropriately challenging and opening eyes to possible alternatives, sometimes inhibited change by putting people's backs up.

The head of steam, which each of the above considerations fuelled in the last years of the twentieth century, has inevitably led to new developments in the way the primary care sector related to the rest of the NHS and to individual patients and local communities.

The new NHS

The 1997 Labour government white paper[4] outlined new responsibilities for the primary care sector. The new responsibilities of the sector were to be underpinned and made safer by the development of new corporate organisations within the sector (PCGs and PCTs in England). These organisations serve a population much larger than the individual practice (commonly more than 100 000) and as they have matured, they have been able to take more responsibility from health authorities. As has been discussed elsewhere, the key change has been the shift in the way resources are allocated through the health service (*see* Figure 7.1).

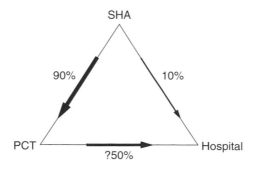

Figure 7.1:   Powerful organisations.

Consideration of this triangle will indicate that primary care is being given major new responsibilities, in exchange for being held to account for the discharge of those responsibilities by the rest of the health service. PCTs will have to account to SHAs, books will have to be open, high trust relationships will matter, continuing support and development, nurturing and facilitation will need to characterise behaviour, if the transfer of resources and power this diagram illustrates is to be safe.

The new 'responsibilities' of the emerging corporate primary care organisations can be illustrated as in Figure 7.2.

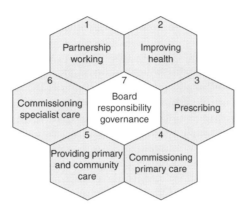

Figure 7.2:   New responsibilities.

If these represent the current agenda for primary care organisations, then Figure 7.3 can be seen as representing some aspects of the development path for PCTs over the next few years. We shall consider each of the current elements making up this agenda before looking at what Choice First and the Feel Good Factor have to offer as illustrations of how the sector might look in a few years' time.

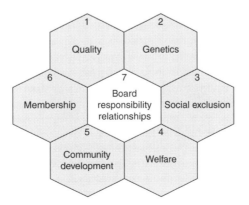

Figure 7.3:   Developing responsibilities.

New responsibilities

Partnership working

In the old NHS and particularly in primary care, practice was monitored and changed through national contract negotiations with little local flexibility. In the internal markets of the 1990s, local flexibilities meant great variation in the quality and provision of primary care services. Primary care trusts are charged with developing an alternative means of improving the quality of care patients receive. This alternative is described as partnership working although this, of course, characterised much that has been good about the primary care sector in the past. Partnership working implies that all the parties involved with an issue sublimate some aspects of their personal power for an agreed, common good. In addition, there is the implication that the partners trust each other, at least to the extent of their commitment to the partnership, and that the parties agree with each other on what they want to achieve and how they are going to do it. In the primary care sector, bringing together the multiplicity of care providers, including independent contractors, social services and the voluntary sector, is an important prerequisite to developing partnership working. Only when they come together to discuss the issues that concern them, and consider how to improve the care that patients receive, can trust start to be built between them and commitment to joint working under a partnership arrangement be developed. The design of PCGs with boards representing nursing, general practice, social services, health service management and the local community started this process and has begun to break down some of the barriers that have existed between providers and between them and other stakeholders.

General practices vary greatly from each other in the approach they have historically taken to:

- service provision
- investment
- team development
- health improvement, etc.

Similarly, the extent to which they have collaborated with, or worked in partnership with, community trust staff, social services and the voluntary sector varies. PCGs have begun to break down some of the barriers to partnership working and through programmes such as the health improvement programme, clinical governance and commissioning, groups have begun to show how partnership working can be effective. At this stage, the extent of trust between the parties, the degree of commitment of resources by the parties and the extent to which they are prepared to give up power for 'the common good' are fairly limited. Over time, the responsibility of the PCTs will be to use partnership working as a vehicle to tackle some of the challenges they face as an organisation, e.g. tackling health inequalities, the inverse care law, social exclusion, etc.

Improving health

While the primary care sector has historically been focused on managing disease, PCTs are also responsible for improving the health of the population. To do this, they will need to assess the health needs of the community, understand the current health status of that community and appreciate the potential for improving the existing health status. In addition, they will need to understand the resource implications involved in addressing health needs and the difficulties that they will face, although many of the disease burdens which faced the NHS in its early years – the acute epidemics, TB, the burden of chronic disability, congenital handicap and disability – are less prevalent now. The twentieth century's epidemics of coronary heart disease, cancer, asthma, obesity and diabetes comprise a disease burden which sets a huge agenda for management by the primary care sector. For PCTs, improving health means not just better management of these and other diseases but also the prevention of the development of disease, the promotion of healthier lifestyles and behaviour through which individual members of the community can develop a greater sense of self-reliance and personal responsibility for their own health. Improving health has to be seen as both a personal responsibility and a community responsibility, with the PCT acting as the fulcrum in balancing the continuing need for disease management with the community's requirement for improved health (*see* Figure 7.4).

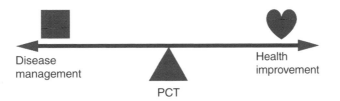

Figure 7.4:   The primary care trust acting as a fulcrum in balancing needs.

Prescribing

As with other specialist, technical management areas, such as human resources, estates, financial management and planning, so clinical areas such as prescribing are responsibilities which many non-clinicians working for PCTs or sitting on their boards will need to understand if they are to discharge their responsibility effectively.

Drugs are relatively expensive, prescribing is the most common clinical intervention in primary care and the quantity of drugs prescribed makes the cost of prescribing a very important issue for the whole health service and all PCTs. The average GP prescribes about £100 000 worth of drugs for his or her patients each year. This means that the average PCT will have a prescribing expenditure of about £10m and, over many years, this expenditure has been rising much faster than the rate of inflation. There are several reasons for this.

1   Drug companies are dynamic powerful organisations which actively market their products and new developments to prescribers, provide the great majority of resources underpinning primary care education and training and are driven by the needs of their shareholders rather than by the policies and requirements of the PCT. Their research and development costs, their global market focus and their capital intensive processes are all expensive.

2   In addition pressure on prescribing budgets from National Service Frameworks (NSFs) and NICE guidance – designed to improve the quality of care patients receive through the NHS – means that prescribers can claim that almost any overspend is justified. Challenging these claims is a risky business for managers and pharmacists.

3   The population is ageing and the elderly need more prescriptions. As more and more older people are cared for outside hospitals, so more of their care has to be paid for from the primary care prescribing budget.

4   Other than through the mechanisms of fundholding and occasionally through the design of PMS contracts, prescribers have not been effectively held to account or made to accept responsibility for their prescribing behaviour. The needs of patients for drugs varies depending on their health status and the behaviour of prescribers varies in ways which have as much to do with their experience and reaction to marketing and management pressures as it has to do with NICE recommendations or evidence based practice.

5   The NHS has failed to get across the message to prescribers over the years, that the more they spend on drugs, the less money will be available for other parts of the healthcare system. The fact that in past years the primary care drug budget was not cash limited and was used by health authorities and hospitals to fund treatments which could not be paid for from hospital budgets, sometimes led to a feeling by prescribers that prescribing costs represented 'monopoly money' rather than real cash. The fact that general practitioners' own take home income, especially if they were dispensing doctors, was dependent on their prescribing behaviour, also made the task of health authority prescribing and medical advisers, when they challenged prescribing behaviour, more difficult. In recent years, health authorities' whole financial performance and balance has been put at risk by burgeoning prescribing costs and they have been forced to pay more and more attention to the requirement for managing these budgets effectively. The employment of medical advisers and pharmacists as prescribing advisers has been their response, but thus far, with limited evidence, they have been able to improve the effectiveness and efficiency of the prescribing system. Pharmacists may know a great deal about medicines and their uses but they know little about pathology, diagnostics, care management and the alternative to drug

prescription which might be appropriate for the management of primary care conditions. As pharmacists, their working experience has been concerned with the supply of medicines, rather than the use of alternative types of therapy such as:

- cognitive behavioural therapy for depression
- physiotherapy for respiratory and orthopaedic problems
- hypnotherapy for psychological problems
- relaxation therapy for stress related distress
- occupational therapy for promoting independence
- counselling for helping individuals gain more insight into, and control over, their lives.

6   Each year, practices are set, and in theory they agree to, a drug budget within which they are expected to manage. Setting the budget is not easy – patients' needs vary with time, practices change and grow, new treatments and changing types of care all conspire to make drug budget setting as much an art as a science. Annual budget cycles, delayed advice from the Department of Health and delays involved in commissioning arrangements (SAFF processes) don't help.

Sadly, because there are limited incentives or disincentives for practices to manage within their budget, many ignore the budget completely. The considerable investment in providing feedback about prescribing performance through the PPA and the provision of prescribing analysis and cost (PACT) data, too often fuel the paper mountain on prescribers' desks rather than changing their prescribing behaviour.

Until adequate incentives are developed to promote and reward high quality effective prescribing, this situation is likely to continue. Nevertheless, in the United Kingdom, prescribers are relatively conservative compared to their counterparts in other Western European or American systems.

We can see (Table 7.1) the scale of the problem which one PCT faces. Serving a population 87 118, their drug budget for the year 2001/2 was £8.557m, meaning an average budget of £98 for every member of the community. Each practice has a drug budget varying between £81.81 and £124.92 per patient. All but one practice are predicted by two-thirds of the way through the year to overspend on their drug budgets by varying amounts between 1% and 20%. As a result, the PCT is expecting an 11% overspend on the drug budget amounting to some £937 416. In order to balance its books, the PCT will need to find this amount from other budgets and inevitably this will have considerable impact on the organisation's ability to discharge its other responsibilities.

For PCTs to begin to address the issues raised by their responsibility for prescribing, they need to:

- understand the prescribing system and the reasons that it works the way it does

Table 7.1: Prescribing performance: Dec 2001

Practice	List	Budget	Budget per patient	Forecast expenditure per patient	Difference	%
D	11 413	1 114 965	97.69	116.40	213 540	19
F	8 124	769 367	94.70	106.91	99 202	13
G	5 600	566 706	101.19	104.15	16 525	3
Go	13 500	1 350 908	100.06	114.99	201 586	15
J	7 308	703 251	96.23	95.86	−2 652	0
K	7 338	746 862	101.78	111.04	67 972	9
R	8 029	773 577	96.35	97.06	5 771	1
P1	1 478	184 639	124.92	143.49	27 435	15
P2	6 500	531 791	81.81	87.28	35 573	7
T	8 707	874 391	100.42	119.06	162 227	19
V	2 984	305 819	102.51	111.93	28 183	9
W	6 137	634 840	103.44	116.81	82 054	13
T	87 118	8 557 116	98.224	108.98	937 416	11

- analyse and understand the behaviour of prescribers, patients and dispensers in detail
- understand the alternatives to current behaviour that exist or might exist
- persuade prescribers and provide incentives for prescribers so that they change their behaviour so as to meet the needs of their patients and the policies and priorities of the PCTs.

This will not be easy and will not happen suddenly. Some 80% of prescribing is of drugs which patients take for many months or years through the 'repeat prescribing system'. Patients will naturally resist changes to their prescription, especially if they feel this is being done for financial rather than clinical quality reasons. Changing patients' repeat prescriptions and the behaviour of prescribers requires a concerted change management programme by PCTs looking at both prescriber and patient perspectives.

PCTs may well also look to including the prescribing budget within a locally agreed practice budget covering premises, staffing, specialist referral, etc., as well as drugs. Experiments through pilot projects such as PMS are currently under way in this area, as are other experiments to look at the electronic supply of medicines and at using pharmacists as medicine managers in primary care. We can anticipate that PCTs will see their responsibility for managing the prescribing budget as a key determinant of their success or failure. Perhaps PCTs might aim to:

- abolish repeat prescribing systems – with all the paper chase, inconvenience to patients, risks of mistakes and inefficient use of staff and doctor time that is involved[5]

- introduce medicine management and advice programmes to promote patient independence and encourage them to understand and take control of their own pathology and its medication
- develop 'clinical pharmacy in primary care' initiatives to promote the efficiency and effectiveness of medication and make better use of the skilled professionals involved
- embrace e-prescribing initiatives so as to make the medicine supply chain not only shorter, but also safer.

At least PCTs might challenge current inequities and inefficiencies by encouraging a rethink and redesign of the system.

Commissioning primary care

As has been indicated in the previous section, the responsibility which PCTs have for the provision of primary care must make them interested in developing new ways of ensuring that the care provided is driven by what is needed by the local community. Some moves away from the centrally imposed national contracts which have underpinned the provision of primary care services up until now can be anticipated. PCTs will want to influence the behaviour of practices and other providers and will want to develop both a partnership approach (*see* above) and an approach which improves the quality of care which patients receive. There must, however, remain some limitations to the freedom of PCTs to totally develop local contracts. Challenging the inverse care law, deprivation, social exclusion and the broader public health agenda must mean that some national priorities and policies remain part of the contract between PCTs and primary care providers. The issues of:

- 'postcode prescribing'
- property price variation
- recruitment and retention of staff difficulties and
- variation in the accessibility, availability and the quality of specialist care, all need to be reflected in a contract between PCTs and providers of primary care services which balances local factors with national perspectives.

As PCTs mature and begin to set their own priorities, in agreement with SHAs, so they will wish to commission care from both secondary and primary care providers to address their particular priorities. In my own PCG, the board has agreed priority areas such as management of drug abuse, teenage services and the development of intermediate care. Although the organisation has been able to initiate some project working in these areas and has worked with the local drug action team (DAT) to develop substance abuse services, its inability to contract with primary care providers to develop new services in these priority areas has constrained its activity. In other areas, priorities such as:

- primary care for refugees
- care of the elderly and nursing in residential care homes
- care of the homeless
- chronic diseases as a result of employment
- problems of rural isolation and falling agricultural incomes

might serve to drive particular PCTs' interests in commissioning appropriate primary care services.

Providing primary and community care

As well as commissioning primary care services, PCTs will also provide primary care services themselves and, in addition, will have inherited responsibilities for the provision of other, more specialist, community services. One of the responsibilities which distinguishes PCTs from PCGs is the employment of staff, who have transferred from previous community trusts. These staff include district nurses and health visitors but also specialist doctors such as paediatricians, community dental practitioners, specialist physiotherapists, occupational therapists, dieticians, chiropodists, etc. They either provide their care as 'first point of contact', i.e. primary care services, or following referral or delegation from primary care, i.e. specialist or secondary care services. Many of the practitioners and services involved have close working relationships with independent contractor primary care services, social services and the voluntary sector and form part of the complex pattern of inter-related and inter-dependent services which previously made up the primary and community care sector.

PCTs will inherit responsibilities for:

- ensuring that the quality of services they directly provide is high
- effectively monitoring practitioner and team performance and
- encouraging service development in the light of evidence, change in the needs of the local community and the needs of practitioners.

Trusts will need to appreciate that as direct providers of this range of services, they will be monitored and have their performance managed by SHAs who will wish to ensure that there are no conflicts of interest between the responsibilities of PCTs as providers and commissioners of care. PCTs will need to consider whether they will continue to provide all the elements that they have inherited, or whether they would wish to commission some elements of care from other providers, be they in primary care or in specialist care. Examples might include primary care nursing where the possibility of developing integrated nursing teams spanning practice nursing, district nursing, health visiting, community psychiatric nursing, learning disabilities nursing, occupational health nursing, school nursing and nursing in residential and nursing care situations might be considered. Presently, these nursing functions are provided by a whole range of providers and PCTs might seek either to provide the whole range themselves or to commission a more integrated approach from an external provider, either in the private sector, voluntary sector or from the existing primary care provider. Alternative arrangements for the provision of other specialist care, such as community paediatrics, occupational health or physiotherapy might also be considered and should include the possibility of commissioning care from specialist providers operating across a wider area than one PCT.

Commissioning specialist care

PCTs have inherited responsibility for commissioning specialist care from health authorities. For the majority of specialist services available at district general hospitals, PCTs will work with other local PCTs, while for more specialist services such as neurosurgery and paediatric intensive care, lead PCTs or regional consortiums are likely to be the commissioning agent. Commissioning is, however, quite a complex and specialist area of activity. The knowledge of current service provision, the experience of how services have developed and their inter-relationships, the understanding of the available measures of performance and the change management skills necessary to adapt current service provision to the needs of the community, are all areas which PCTs will need to address. The transfer of staff from health authorities, with public health and commissioning experience, will be important to PCTs but, in addition, they need to add value from within their experience, if they are to be more successful than health authorities. This added value must come from the utilisation of the clinical experience of primary care providers within the PCTs. Patients' experience of specialist care influences how primary care practitioners such as GPs behave – they will refer to one consultant rather than another, and use one service for one reason and another in other circumstances. Using this wealth of experience, built up over many years and constantly refined by the experience of patients, should enable the commissioning process to be more effective. Incorporating the clinician's perspective in commissioning arrangements was shown to be useful on a micro-scale during the years of GP fundholding[2] and now needs to be further developed by PCTs. The possibility of reconfiguring the way clinical services are put together across organisational and care sector boundaries will need to be considered, as will issues such as the following.

- Common medical records across primary and secondary care.
- Electronic communications for laboratories and referral letters.

Box 7.1:   Case study – Di's baby

Di is 36, 17 weeks into her second pregnancy which has been long delayed because her daughter Anne, who had cystic fibrosis, needed all her care until she sadly died last year.

Her antenatal care is largely provided by Dee, her community midwife – employed by the acute trust and following her mums throughout their pregnancy, across organisational boundaries, a real ally against the often threatening complexity of the NHS 'system'. Di's CF tests have all come back normal, but on Friday she gets a call from her GP. Dee is on holiday and there is a problem with Di's blood tests. The GP's computerised results service has alerted him to her raised AFP – she will need to see a specialist and have further tests. Di spends a very anxious week until she meets Mr Dass, the obstetrician. He doesn't know about Anne, only that Di's results and scan suggest spina bifida.

He recommends that Di consider a termination – she opts for it and by the time Dee returns it is all over.

The system worked – communications happened and technical, high quality care was provided. However, things could and should have been better – all the team and Di know that. The task for PCTs is to design the system to ensure that:

- Dee's holiday didn't leave Di high and dry
- the GP was there for Di when she saw Mr Dass, had her scan and made her decision
- the records ensured Mr Dass knew Di's background
- the system didn't leave Di anxious and alone for the week between initial result and appointment.

So often, current systems work because committed individuals make them work, rather than because they are designed to work.

- Reconfiguring accident and emergency care by looking at the roles and responsibilities of walk-in centres, NHS Direct, ambulance services and A&E.
- Direct booking for waiting lists in general surgery, orthopaedics, ENT, etc. to avoid the inefficiencies of outpatient waiting lists and the uncertainty of not knowing how long you, as a patient, are going to have to wait for effective treatment.
- Integrating clinical care between the home and hospital so that general medical practice, medicine management expertise and nursing skills can be used more flexibly between the ward and the home environment when clinically indicated.

- Examples such as midwives and dialysis nurses following patients into and out of hospital can also be used to improve quality in cancer care, genetic care, diabetes, etc.
- Specialist outreach nurses and the possibility of clinical assistant or specialist primary care practitioners working both within and outside hospital should be considered. This additional clinical input into commissioning should help to clarify the added advantage of PCTs as 'clinical managers', a step on from 'general managers' with clinical support, which was the approach taken by health authorities. The requirement will be for PCTs to equip their clinicians to support commissioning, and resource the process adequately so that the clinicians understand how they can add value to the process without feeling that they are overwhelmed by the data and financial issues. Enabling primary care clinicians to operate outside their traditional sphere of influence, challenge the behaviour of specialist units, and have the mental flexibility to consider how the needs of their patients make them act differently, will require considerable investment in developing their knowledge base and change management skills. Nevertheless, the benefits from this approach were considerable under fundholding and should provide a rich source of leverage for PCTs.

Board responsibility 'governance'

The issues of corporate governance for primary care have been described earlier in this book (*see* Chapter 2). PCTs, as with other health service trusts, have corporate governance responsibilities for discharging effectively the powers that they have inherited. What they will not have is textbooks telling them how to develop the required corporate governance approach within the primary care sector, where in the past the governing arrangements were very different. Partnership agreements between independent contractors did not deal with issues of openness, accountability, public involvement, probity and scrutiny in the way that PCTs will need to establish themselves. Helping board members, whose experience has been within the primary care sector in the past, to understand the needs for, and benefits of, appropriate corporate governance will be an early task, which should not be underestimated. PCGs have sometimes struggled with issues of openness and public debate, and cannot be expected to give up their heritage of confidential, professional partnerships overnight. The importance of the non-executive role in PCTs should not be underestimated. In the past, the primary care sector has been driven by executive practitioners who are capitalisers of the sector, employers of staff, directors of their practices and shop floor workers. In the past they have not been posed the challenge which non-executive directors will pose in the future. Patients have, by and large, not had the power to challenge practice policies. Non-executives on PCT boards will need to challenge primary care behaviour and PCT executive functions, if the

PCTs are to demonstrate effective corporate governance and be responsive to the needs of the community rather than the needs of practitioners.

Developing responsibilities

As primary care organisations mature, they are beginning to move on from the operational management or 'anatomy' of the primary care sector and to look at some of the issues for which they are accountable and which span across the above areas of responsibility, serve to relate them to each other and determine where change and investment might have benefit throughout the system. In this context, we can consider that primary care organisations are being encouraged to foster, and are developing, a more physiological approach to management of the primary care system, with all the homeostatic mechanisms, feedback loops, balancing mechanisms, etc. which we have discussed in earlier chapters. This supportive and facilitative approach to development of the sector contrasts with the approach in earlier years which was characterised by the following issues.

- Rigid national contracts and regulations whose function was to constrain innovation and promote an even, equitable and fair distribution of resource, i.e. a Ford Cortina approach.
- Administration of the sector through a succession of organisations, such as executive councils, family practitioner committees, family health services authorities, health commissions and, lastly, LHAs. Their role was to administer the functioning of the sector through implementing national agreements and contracts, rather than managing the sector, i.e. facilitating development and change in response to changing local circumstance.
- The focus was *within* the primary care sector and particularly within general practice rather than looking at all of the various elements of the primary care sector together, including other local independent contractors, community trust staff working with primary care, social services staff working with primary care, voluntary sector workers, etc. and without looking at the provision of care across organisational boundaries. Due consideration was seldom given to the pathways of care that patients experience, such as between hospital and home, but also including hospices, nursing and residential care homes, community hospitals, day centres, etc.

The consequences of this style of management have been to promote a rigid, inflexible, centrally driven, patronising and paternalistic style of healthcare delivery – but also one that is fairly efficient, fair, cost effective and enjoys the public's confidence.

As circumstances and society change, so this type of administration of the primary care sector has been seen to be in need of further development if it is to address current issues of concern to the community. This is not to deny the

importance of national priorities, centrally set standards, efficient administration and the heritage of long-term support and of high quality care provision.

Quality

As primary care organisations have begun to look at the care that is provided
within their area, they are beginning to try and improve the quality of care
which patients receive. Quality is a multi-faceted concept and as illustrated in
Figure 7.5 can be considered under many different headings.

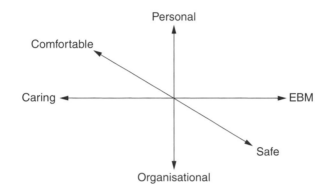

Figure 7.5:   Quality of care considered under different headings.

PCTs have responsibility for ensuring and promoting the quality of care provided
to their local population and are having to consider the issue by reflecting on all
the facets involved. *Clinical governance* is the umbrella term under which the
aspects of clinical quality are being addressed. Existing approaches such as:

- education and training
- audit including medical, clinical, significant event and financial
- research and development
- public involvement
- risk management
- team development

are being supported through investment in:

- protected time for education and development, such as the TARGET scheme
  in Doncaster
- supported team and practice development time
- the development of quality assurance programmes such as the Health Quality
  Service, the RCGP Quality and Practice programme, Commission for Health
  Improvement, etc.
- encouragement of significant event audit[6]

- the development of personal development plans and practice development plans, encouraging a development path for individuals and organisations which will equip them better to meet their own needs and the needs of their local population
- the valuing of the primary care workforce through their inclusion in occupational health schemes, staff pension arrangements and local committees and working groups, striving to interpret national priorities, such as NSFs, in the light of local circumstance.

As PCTs advance they will need to develop additional tools and levers for promoting quality. They will consider the extent to which they wish to maintain and promote the primary care heritage of continuing personal, biographical care, or move further towards quality defined through an evidence based approach to quality which is safe, efficient and effective and whether the two are mutually exclusive, or inter-dependent. There is no doubt that central national quality assurance mechanisms to deal with poor performance, such as local performance review quartets, the National Clinical Assessment Authority and revised GMC/UKCC arrangements with PREP, revalidation, re-accreditation, the ending of PGEA, etc. are important supportive steps to re-defining professional behaviour in a way which is more responsive and fit to meet the needs of the community.

Genetics

Developments in molecular biology and genetics over the last 40 years have built on our understanding of the structure of DNA and have culminated in the completion of the human gene project. Understanding the anatomy of DNA, genes, RNA, etc. now opens up the possibility of beginning to understand the physiology and biochemistry of genetics. Until now, the impact of genetics in primary care has been limited to the relatively rare inherited diseases which pose a significant burden to those suffering from them and to the local support services, but are not so frequent or so much of a burden to the health service that it has focused a great deal of attention on them. Diseases such as muscular dystrophy (sex linked), cystic fibrosis (autosomal recessive) and Huntington's chorea (autosomal dominant), form the genetic disease burden which the NHS has focused on. The help needed by people suffering from these genetic illnesses has been found through all the major specialist services and been co-ordinated by the regional clinical genetics centres and their associated laboratories. Primary care has had little involvement with genetic illness until now. Primary care has concentrated on illnesses that are largely environmental and have been little affected by the impact of inheritance.

Nevertheless, we are all affected by our inheritance. Our genes *are* our heritage and they do affect many aspects of our lives. In addition, they are our contribution to future generations, our children and their children inherit them along with our property, wealth, attitudes and values (at least those left after the tax man has had his share). As we understand more about the anatomy, physiology and biochemistry of our genetic inheritance, so we can begin to see how it affects our susceptibility to disease, the likelihood that we will respond to treatment and the changes we might make to our lifestyle to the benefit of ourselves, our families and future generations. As PCTs are developing, they need to take seriously the impact of inheritance and genetic medicine on the services they provide and commission.

First steps into the world of genetic medicine for primary care have come from the identification of susceptibility genes for breast and ovarian cancer. Because of the common occurrence of these cancers generally and, therefore, within families, so the identification of susceptibility genes has caused some difficulties. Because primary care practitioners have received little training in genetic medicine, they will naturally refer to specialist clinical genetic services when they feel that they are not equipped to offer appropriate advice. Only a small proportion (less than 5%) of patients with breast or ovarian cancer develop these as a result of carrying the susceptibility genes,[7] but the perfectly understandable concern of relatives and patients and the weakness of primary care as a gatekeeper in this area has meant a considerable burden for clinical genetic services.

Other inherited traits which increase the risk of disease also raise difficult ethical and long-term management questions for those affected and their advisers in the primary care team. Familial hypercholesterolaemia is but one example of a metabolic consequence of inheritance, which increases the risk of early, severe, ischaemic heart disease.

In addition, each and every one of us has a varying, but quantifiable and real, genetic burden as a result of inheriting a unique combination of the 30 000 genes which make up our heritage.

A new area which primary care practitioners will need to become familiar with is pharmacogenetics. It has been known for many years that our inherited acetylation status can determine how we react to isoniazid (used in the treatment of TB). We can now appreciate with the development of genetic finger printing – particularly involving single nucleotide polymorphisms (SNIP) – that the better targeting of therapy to those most likely to benefit is under rapid development. These developments will mean that many of the local population will need to be tested and their SNIP profiles determined, before therapy is initiated. It may well be that SNIP maps will help individuals make decisions about marriage and having a family as we can anticipate them equipping individual citizens to make more informed choices about their own and their children's genetic risk.

Some communities are already experiencing the consequences of inherited disease to a greater extent than others. Communities from the eastern Mediterranean with a high prevalence of thalassaemia and those African and West Indian communities with a large haemoglobinopathy burden are examples where informed decision making by families, carriers and those affected, with the support of their specialist and primary care advisers, already plays a significant part in primary care provision. In other areas, testing for chromosome abnormalities in early pregnancy has posed difficulties for midwives and other primary care practitioners as their education and training have failed to equip them adequately for the roles and responsibilities they face.

PCTs, in developing the capacity within their community and workforce to address the issues raised by genetic medicine, will require support from the regional clinical genetics specialist services and will need to develop a system which is flexible enough to deal with the needs of the local community, while equipping the workforce to understand and interpret this rapidly developing and potentially highly empowering technology.

The requirement is likely to be for an education and training programme to equip:

- large numbers of practitioners – nurses, doctors, counsellors, pharmacists, midwives, etc. to be effective gatekeepers and practitioners of genetic medicine for their local population
- a smaller number of practitioners in each community to support the development and implementation of genetic medicine
- a lead clinician in each PCT to work with local practice and the clinical genetic specialist services to co-ordinate and act as a more informed gatekeeper between primary care genetic medicine and regional specialist clinical genetic services. PCTs will need to develop this systematic approach to developing knowledge, promoting efficient utilisation of scarce specialist resources and providing the capacity and flexibility of response to deal with a rapidly changing and evolving area of care.

We should not forget that decision making in genetic medicine can have implications, not just for the individual, but for their family and succeeding generations. Making decisions about genetic issues is difficult for individuals and they need support and skilled counselling to deal with the moral and ethical issues they confront. PCTs will need to be sensitive to the values and beliefs of their local communities and go to great lengths to avoid any suspicion that they, and the community they represent, have any kind of a party line on any genetic issue or wish to pressurise individuals to make decisions in the wider communities' interest rather than their own.

Box 7.2:   Case study – Cystic fibrosis

Jane and David were only children and had one daughter, Anne, who was diagnosed as having cystic fibrosis. She was largely cared for at home with the support of the primary care team but had many admissions and visits to local and regional specialist services. Sadly, as with many people with cystic fibrosis, she developed severe lung problems and died at the age of nine. Because of Anne's illness, her parents had decided not to have further children, but soon after her death, the possibility of genetic testing in early pregnancy became available and they decided to try again. Chorionic villous sampling in early pregnancy showed the new baby to be a carrier but not affected, much to her parent's joy and relief. Sadly, 10 days later, the news that the baby had a chromosome abnormality came as a crushing blow which, following time and supportive counselling, led to their decision to terminate the pregnancy. The following year, Jane again fell pregnant and again went through testing. Happily this time, all was well and Rosie has been the apple of her parents' eye ever since.

This story is not unique, the issues raised are faced by every primary care team each year and by thousands of families scattered across the country. They require skilled and expert handling by a combination of specialist services and a primary care team, trained, educated and informed to support families through such difficult times.

Social exclusion

PCTs have responsibility for promoting the health of the whole of their local population. Sadly, the social revolution of the twentieth century has not led to an improved health status of the whole population. Despite increasing affluence, the NHS has failed to tackle the inverse care, and the disenfranchised minority groups are as much in need now as they ever have been of support and help from PCTs. Such groups, whose needs are great, often receive little publicity and attention and often have least power to affect the policies and decision-making forums of health authorities and trusts.

In establishing the Social Exclusion Unit at the Cabinet Office, the post-1997 Labour government recognised that such excluded minorities required a special and focused attention across government departments if effective interventions were to be found to address their needs and improve the overall health of the whole community.

Those highlighted as having special needs were:

- lager louts and lasses – the disaffected adolescents
- girls affected by teenage pregnancy, which sadly is more common in the United Kingdom than in many developed countries and a cause of distress not only to the individuals concerned but to their wider family and friends
- people addicted to drugs and alcohol and those who suffer the direct and indirect consequences of their dependency
- people with learning disabilities whose needs and families' needs are often complex and span education, social services, health and employment
- people with severe and enduring mental health problems who now increasingly live in community homes or with their families but who often find themselves excluded from community activities

- the isolated, vulnerable and frequently frail elderly, particularly those with mental health problems
- people in institutional care – be that in prisons or long stay health institutions which may become communities in themselves, but which frequently exclude themselves and their members from accessing the opportunities and benefits available to the broader community.

The task then for PCTs is to assume responsibility for the whole of their community and ensure that their plans address the needs of these excluded minorities.

Box 7.3:   Case study

The Grange was a community established in the 1960s for adults with learning disabilities. Several houses scattered around a small village green in the most rural part of the PCT were home to some 70 adults and 50 carers who have devoted their lives to the development of the community and the care of the residents. Young volunteers and local supporters supplemented the care in what was a happy and vibrant small community. A local general practice had, for many years, taken responsibility for the care of this community but dental and ophthalmic support frequently had to be hospital based and the specialist care of residents with mental health, skin, epilepsy and other chronic diseases had sometimes been sub-optimal.

Welfare

The holistic heritage of primary care has meant that it is always recognised that health is much more than just the absence of disease. The social and spiritual welfare of individuals is as important to their happiness and to them leading fulfilled lives as is effective treatment of their physical needs. If PCTs and the rest of the health service focus all their attention on the prevention, diagnosis and management of disease, then they fail to address the full range of health needs of the community and the individuals who make it up.

Partnership working with social services (*see* above) will need to become the precursor of a joint approach between PCTs and social services to promote the welfare of the local community. Issues such as lone parenting, serial monogamy and the problems of the isolated single elderly highlight the need not only to care through addressing their health needs but also through supporting them and helping them meet their social needs. PCTs might need to encourage mother and toddler groups, relationship counselling services, meals on wheels and befriending services for the elderly and through such interventions to encourage health promoting behaviour, disease prevention strategies and a greater sense of empowerment for individuals through their taking a greater responsibility for their own health and welfare.

Community development

If PCTs are to effectively challenge the inverse care law and promote the health of the whole community, then they will need to work closely with those who had previous worked in the field of community development. The United Kingdom has a proud heritage in the voluntary sector in this area, through groups which range from the boy scouts to the Red Cross, from volunteer driving and transport services to supporting youth clubs or shopping services for the elderly. This has provided a rich heritage of voluntary contribution to the community which PCTs will need to harness and develop to a much greater extent than has been apparent in the past. While the autonomy, flexibility and focus of each service has to be respected and supported if the commitment of volunteers is to continue to evolve, PCTs will need to ensure that the socially excluded and less attractive groups are not ignored. Services for the mentally infirm elderly and those with learning disabilities, for example, will need to be encouraged.

Membership

If PCTs are to address these areas of responsibility, then they will need to find ways to encourage individual members of the community to feel that the PCT is their trust. Individuals will need to feel that the trust is acting on their behalf, is helping to address their health and welfare needs and is developing, commissioning and providing health services which are relevant to them. If the PCT is to achieve these aims, it has to be able to listen to the views of the individuals making up its community and to ensure that those views are given due weight in developing the policies and plans of the organisation. The introduction of non-executive lay members to the boards of PCTs marks an important advance in developing a more open and accountable approach to corporate governance than has been the heritage of primary care in the past but, as time moves on, it may well be that PCTs need to strengthen their commitment and the relationship with their local communities to achieve their objectives. Traditional open meetings and forums for public participation in the decision-making processes of health authorities and trusts have frequently failed to attract widespread involvement, but nevertheless, holding such meetings and holding board meetings in public are important preliminary steps to demonstrating the place PCTs have in the community. PCTs will, however, need to learn lessons from other community based organisations, such as housing associations and the voluntary sector, if they are to ensure that they have the support and commitment of individuals and the whole community for the future. They will need to balance such support and commitment against their requirements to be part of the NHS, which requires the PCT to address important national priorities such as financial balance, waiting lists, cancer and coronary heart disease.

Learning lessons from housing associations and the voluntary sector could mean establishing locality forums where individuals and community groups can contribute to the policy development and implementation of the PCT, or the development and support of committees to address particular health issues within the community – rather as the local scout group may be run by a committee of parents, so local services for the frail elderly might involve programmes developed by local committees drawn from their family and friends.

Box 7.4: Case study – A difficult decision at the PCT board

Mary had been diagnosed as having ME – or chronic fatigue syndrome. After several years she has fallen out with the local consultant in rehabilitation and his team. She wanted referral for inpatient treatment at a national centre specialising in the condition, but there is little evidence that this will help her.

Her GP agrees to refer her, if the PCT will support and pay the costs – some £20 000 for the inpatient stay followed by further ongoing supportive therapy. The PCT refuses to support the referral, on the basis of advice that there is not enough evidence that the treatment will help Mary, but she appeals and gets support from the ME association, her MP and the national centre's consultant. Eventually she takes the PCT to judicial review – followed by a trip to Europe fighting for her 'human rights'. The PCT loses, not because it was wrong nor because of new evidence showing the treatment would help, but because the PCT hadn't correctly followed due process allowing Mary to be sufficiently involved at all stages.

In this and other ways, PCTs will emerge as organisations which address the health needs of their local community, either through direct provision or through commissioning services. These then will become organisations which are to a greater or lesser extent driven by the needs of their local communities. The power which individuals have over the organisation, the extent to which the PCT board is accountable and responsive to the views, aspirations and needs of the local community will only evolve over time and will always, of course, have to be balanced by the board's accountability to SHAs and the rest of the health service. Nevertheless, the concept that PCTs might be, at least in part, driven by the needs of the local community, raises the interesting issue of whether they could be considered membership organisations and develop the kind of infrastructure and procedures to support that process of empowering individual members and fostering their commitment.

Every individual in the community has an SP4 (NHS Medical Card). These pre-date the NHS and before the days of the NHS entitled holders of the card to receive free healthcare from their panel doctor. The right to free treatment was extended to the whole community within the NHS and it could be said that the

NHS medical card is really the membership card to the NHS. Patients will still often bring their card when they access health services and indeed are encouraged to by the instructions on the card. The card also enables individuals to change their doctor and explains how to complain about the services they receive. In some ways, this card describes individuals' entitlements under the NHS and defines their rights and responsibilities. The development of the Patients' Charter in the 1980s/1990s was another example of delineating the relationship between individuals and the NHS. Older, pre-Second World War medical cards were sometimes even more explicit in describing the rights and responsibilities of membership and it may be that PCTs will need to build on the heritage of patient charters, medical cards, etc. to more clearly delineate what individuals can expect from the service and what the service can expect from individuals.

Board responsibility relationships

In an earlier section, we looked at the PCT board's responsibilities for governance and this is an important prerequisite of the rest of the health service to the community having confidence in the PCT board and demonstrating that it is safe for the taxpayer and the community to trust the board with the power and resources necessary for it to deliver all its responsibilities. In this section, we consider how the responsibilities of the PCT board are developing beyond the safety net of good governance. We can see from the above description of the board's developing responsibilities that they are mostly addressed through the relationships the PCT has rather than through any direct action of the PCT itself. These relationships include partnership working on the basis of trust and agreed programmes of work with a range of agencies in the local authority, statutory, private and voluntary sectors.

However, PCTs are likely to need to use a range of relationship types if they are to address all their responsibilities. The purchaser/provider relationship which developed under the internal market in the 1980/1990s may again become appropriate for PCTs who commission care from the private sector, e.g. private hospitals, to tackle waiting lists or even international patient care as has recently been tried with hospitals in northern France.

As described above, PCTs will also need to develop mutually supportive relationships to work with the voluntary sector, where, because of their particular bias and special interests, the PCT will want to support their activities without the formal accountability and governance arrangements involved with partnership or purchaser–provider relationships.

The relationship with individual members of the local community, be they members of the PCT or local citizens, has also been described above and will be an important element in establishing a full range of relationships through which the PCT will deliver on its responsibilities. PCTs will only be successful if they manage to balance the interests of their local community with those of the national community and if they do this through relationships which are positive, supportive and constructive and which are designed to improve the quality of care individuals receive via the PCT.

Feel Good Factor and Choice First

Consider how the current and developing responsibilities of PCTs will complement or contradict the responsibilities of primary care organisations in the two futures.

Choice First

The responsibilities which the board of First Call face are illustrated in Figure 7.6.

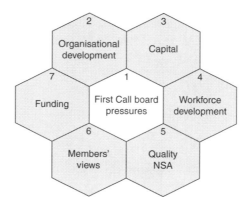

Figure 7.6:   Responsibilities of the board of First Call.

As a 'not for profit' private sector organisation, First Call is under pressure to adequately capitalise on and develop its services. The pressure to expand so that economies of scale can be maximised is no different to the choice facing small PCTs, but the evolution of information and technology has meant that larger populations and memberships can be looked after without losing the organisation's sensitivity to the needs and aspirations of its members.

As with the culture of PCTs, First Call is focused on quality improvement and workforce development. The National Standards Agency may have replaced the Audit Commission, NICE and the Commission for Health Improvement, but the focus on quality assurance of the services First Call provides and demonstrating that quality explicitly to the membership is a powerful marketing tool for the organisation. Developing the workforce, both to ensure recruitment and retention of all staff groups, and to ensure they remain committed to the organisation and motivated to provide the highest quality healthcare to the membership remains, whereas PCTs face the challenge of integrating the various historic funding streams which have resourced workforce development, e.g. non-medical education and training, medical and dental education levy and FHSA/practice training budgets. PCTs are faced with a myriad of education systems with accountabilities to Royal Colleges, university departments, health authorities and professional associations. The First Call board has developed a co-ordinated and cohesive workforce development programme which has removed many of the barriers which have prevented talented individuals fulfilling their career aspirations in primary care in the past.

As an organisation, which is dependent on its membership, the board of First Call is much more sensitive to their views and requirements than early PCTs are. But the extent to which users feel involved is still relatively limited as this is a large private sector organisation where the views of individual shareholders are likely to be as marginal as they are in any private company. Institutional shareholders and the funders, e.g. insurance companies and merchant banks, are likely to be influential.

Box 7.5:   Case study – A difficult decision at First Call's board

Mary's case (Box 7.4) is repeated as an issue for First Call's board – they make the same decision as the PCT, based on evidence of effectiveness and again are taken to judicial review and Europe. They win their case because they had followed due process. Mary was a member, had voted the board in, managed her PIA, insured for extra treatment, but the insurer excluded inpatient treatment.

Nevertheless, the development of personal investment accounts through which individual members of First Call control part of the resource necessary to fund their care, means that the views of individual members and access to their PIAs are important to the board of First Call. The possibility that voluntary effort might increase the value of an individual's personal investment account can be seen to complement the heritage of voluntary activity and its development in PCTs as discussed above, while the issue of caring for those with lifelong disability and inherited disease remains problematic. First Call would seem to be an organisation which will do well if its membership is healthy and only suffers acute short-term illness but may struggle if it is faced with dealing with significant issues raised by social exclusion, lifelong disability and chronic disease. The funding of care of the elderly, institutional care and of the kind of personal and family care discussed in the genetic section will be something for which Choice First will have to develop strict quality standards and be externally monitored against.

The Feel Good Factor

The committee, which supervises the Healthy Living Bureau, remains accountable to regional and central government for its use of the resources which fund the services provided. The responsibilities, which the committee might concentrate on, are illustrated in Figure 7.7.

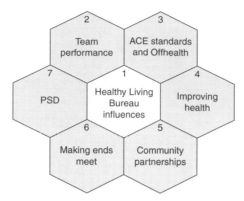

Figure 7.7:   Responsibilities that the committee of the Healthy Living Bureau might concentrate on.

But it is the ethos and way of working of the committee which characterises this future and which can be seen as an extension of some of the developing responsibilities of current PCTs. This is an organisation which relies on community spirit and on the commitment and support of the local community for its success. The Bureau's committee has to work through 'influence' rather than using the levers of performance management, partnership or support and facilitation. Being directly elected, it must ensure that it has the confidence of its voters and this acts as a constraining force in inhibiting the Bureau from rocking the boat. Nevertheless, the ethos is community spirit and there is a considerable pressure on deviant individuals to conform – to stop smoking, drinking while driving, or allowing themselves to become unfit. Influencing and promoting this ethos is an important function of the committee, so as to encourage individuals' personal responsibility for their own health and reduce demand on the services that they provide.

Box 7.6:   Case study – A difficult decision for the Bureau

Mary's case (Box 7.4) is considered by the committee, which supports her inpatient treatment but only if she can demonstrate that she has sufficient voluntary carer input at home to help her rehabilitation. She is pressurised by the parish council and local self-care group to stop smoking, stop abusing the committee and return to the local consultant's care. She agrees to further local treatment but is not happy. Eventually she and her family find the money for private inpatient care, but it makes little difference. The following year the committee pays for her and a carer to go to Bath for a therapeutic week and she returns much happier.

As with current PCTs, the committee has responsibility for care of standards and indeed has a professional standards director (PSD), whose task is quality assurance and ensuring that the accreditation for clinical effectiveness (ACE) standards and the requirements of the regulator (Offhealth) are addressed. This can be seen as an extension of the current clinical governance work of PCTs and their developing responsibilities for quality assurance and implementing evidence based medicines.

Rigid professional boundaries have been channelled in the Healthy Living Bureau to the care and support provided by healthcare teams. It is team performance and the quality of care they provide and individuals receive which defines the quality of care and the teams are monitored against these standards. Individual professional paradigms have largely been sublimated to teamworking although specialist roles within the teams and between teams remain important. In this situation, the care of those with chronic disease or disability, the issues raised by genetic medicine and the issues raised by social exclusion receive more emphasis than the issues raised by needful acute care and disease prevention.

The Healthy Living Bureau, therefore, works by influencing: (i) the environment within which care is provided; (ii) the behaviour of the teams which provide care; and (iii) the behaviour of individuals within the community towards living a healthier lifestyle and constraining their need for healthcare intervention.

Conclusions

These then are some of the responsibilities of the new and rapidly maturing corporate primary care organisations – PCTs in England and their equivalent in Scotland, Wales and Northern Ireland. While concentrating on the challenges and responsibilities that the organisation's boards are facing, can anticipate facing and might expect to face in the two alternative futures, delineated by the *Tomorrow's World* project, we have to appreciate some of the common themes that emerge.

- An emphasis on the quality of care patients receive in the community served by the organisation, through further development of clinical governance at both individual and team levels, with the additional component of quality assurance at an organisational level, either through further development of CHI-NICE-Revalidation-HQS mechanisms or by realigned agencies covering similar responsibilities.
- Closer attention to the relationships between the primary care organisation and its constituent provider practices, etc. and to its care partners from local authority, private and voluntary sectors, with a range of working arrangements between them to support them in jointly meeting the challenges posed by health and broader welfare problems.

- Development of the relationship between the primary care organisation (PCO) and the individual citizens that make up the community served by the PCO. The realisation that it is only through the consent, support and active participation of individual citizens that the ethos of organisations can move from being the management of disease to being the support and development of health within the community. This focus on promoting individual personal responsibility for health with both its genetic and environmental constituents is reflected in the design of the Feel Good Factor as a membership organisation and Choice First as an organisation funded by personal investment accounts and capitalised by its shareholders.

- These organisations have, through sound corporate governance arrangements, demonstrated their trustworthiness and ability to improve the efficiency of healthcare delivery. As a result, they have become responsible for commissioning almost all services and control the vast majority of healthcare resources. Some will have chosen to provide directly an extended range of services, such as rehabilitation, mental health, care of the elderly, etc., while others might have chosen to commission these from other providers, be they in the public, private or voluntary sectors. The key theme is that the PCO has operated in a 'high trust' environment, demonstrated its effective governance arrangements and been trusted by the community with the resources necessary to redesign the patterns of care patients receive: to challenge the centrally planned bureaucratic, under-resourced NHS at the end of the twentieth century; to move on from the feeling that the service was organised around the needs and aspirations of the care providers, be they hospitals or primary care teams, to provide a service which is driven by the needs of individual citizens and the community.

References

1 Huntingdon J (1995) *Managing the Practice: whose business?* King's Fund, London.
2 Audit Commission (1996) *What the Doctor Ordered.* Audit Commission, London.
3 Tudor-Hart J (1998) *A New Kind of Doctor.* Merlin Press, London.
4 Department of Health (1997) *The New NHS: modern, dependable.* DoH White Paper, London.
5 Neary J (2002) Clinical medication review by pharmacists would improve care. *BMJ.* **324**: 548.
6 Department of Health (2000) *An Organisation with a Memory.* DoH, London.
7 Emery J and Hayflick S (2001) The challenge of integrating genetic medicine into primary care. *BMJ.* **322**: 1027–30.

CHAPTER 8

Toolkit for delivery

Previous chapters have dealt with the forces moulding the primary care sector and how they relate to each, the dynamics or physiology of those relationships and the way they are changing over time. We have considered the heritage and how this has influenced the values, attitudes and beliefs of those involved with the development of the primary care sector and the delivery of care through it and by it to its patients, clients and users and the broader community. We have considered why those involved in the sector behave the way they do based on their varying views, roles, responsibilities and relationships. In Chapter 7 we looked at the way such responsibilities are evolving both at the interface between the individual patient/user and his or her primary care practitioner, and at the community, PCO/team interface.

These considerations have dealt with the issues of *why* the primary care sector has been developing the way it has and *how* the design of the primary care sector and practice within the sector has been changing and evolving.

In this chapter we will be consider *what* tools are being used within the primary care sector and by the broader NHS to drive that change and evolution in design and practice. While these tools are often considered in isolation from each other, in this chapter I shall emphasise that they all form constituent parts of the toolkit. Any workman's toolkit – be he a carpenter or a surgeon – contains an array of tools which are seldom used singly. Each has its own purpose, be it a scalpel for cutting through skin or a hammer for banging in nails, but used together they can transform life and the world. This toolkit is:

- adapting practice and organisation within the primary care sector to meet the requirements of modern society
- reflecting the demands which have moved on following the social and industrial revolutions of the nineteenth and twentieth centuries to meet the requirements of the twenty-first century for:
  - quality assurance
  - power sharing
  - good governance
  - personal responsibility.

They all form part of the *community* revolution which we will be considering in the next chapter.

This chapter is therefore about *leverage*. It is about channelling the power of the primary care sector so that it delivers the kind of care which is needed by the individuals and communities that it serves.

It is important to appreciate that the leverage that we are considering is not being applied in a vacuum. The primary care sector has a proud heritage which has always responded and adapted as a result of the forces acting on it, e.g. the development of community pharmacy during the industrial and social revolutions, the growth and sub-specialisation of nursing as well as the development and power of the medical model. Throughout this evolution the sector's development has relied on the implicit trust between individuals seeking healthcare advice and treatment, and those that they consult. The respect, trust and faith which have underpinned these core relationships have meant that the community has allowed the primary care sector a great deal of freedom to evolve and develop without the explicit and overt accountability for the quality of service it provides, and the use of the community's resources. Openness and accountability, responsiveness to consumer views, participation and partnership working are now challenging that heritage of implicit trust, respect and faith.

Examples over recent years such as Beverley Allitt in nursing, Harold Shipman in general practice and other cases which have received wide publicity in the media may well be exceptional cases, but do have an effect on the confidence that individuals and the community have in clinical practice.[1,2] We shall now consider, in more detail, some of the tools which PCTs will need to use synergistically to improve the quality of care patients receive.

Box 8.1:   Case study – PCT's response to Harold Shipman

Following the Baker committee's audit of HS's clinical practice[3] the PCT considered its recommendations and the local implications of them. The recommendations were discussed at the clinical governance group, reviewed at the PEC and the resulting policies endorsed by the board. The board reflected that action was important to reinforce the trust the community had in its general practitioners, even though everyone recognised that HS's case was exceptional – he was a murderer who happened to be a GP, not a poorly performing doctor.

Taking the recommendations in order.

1 Systems for the monitoring of general practitioners should be reviewed and extended to include routine monitoring of death rates, and improved methods for the review of prescribing of controlled drugs and the quality of medical records.
   – To be monitored by the PCT via the practice managers' group, MIQUEST data enquiries and by questioning at practice clinical governance visits.
2 A system for collecting information about the number of deaths of patients of, and MCCDs issued by, general practitioners should be investigated, and a practical system introduced as soon as possible.
   – Action by government (DoH) awaited. In the meantime, review of MCCD counterslips as part of practice CG reviews.

3   In a revised certification system, brief information about the circum-
    stances of death and the patient's clinical history should be recorded
    both in the case of cremation and burials.
    –   Action by government awaited.
4   The procedure for revalidation of general practitioners should include
    an assessment of appropriate samples of a general practitioner's records.
    –   Appraisal, assessment and revalidation programmes under develop-
        ment centrally
5   The policy of offering to return records to general practitioners after the
    expiry of the period of storage by health authorities should be reviewed.
    If general practitioners are allowed to retain records, arrangements
    for their secure storage should be established, and provision for their
    eventual disposal agreed.
    –   Local agreement to cease offering return of records.
6   An effective system for inspection of general practitioners' controlled
    drugs registers should be introduced.
    –   The PCT advised all practitioners to review their arrangements and
        encouraged them to centralise their registers as practice registers.
        The PCT agreed that review of such registers should form part of
        clinical governance reviews.
7   General practitioners should record batch numbers in clinical records
    when they personally administer controlled drugs and batch num-
    bers should be included in the controlled drugs registers of general
    practitioners and pharmacists.
    –   PCT recommendation to practitioners.

MESSAGE: The PCT supports a systematic approach to learning lessons
from events and sees its prime responsibility as ensuring high quality care
of patients. This requires a more open approach to quality assurance so as
to reinforce the confidence that patients and the community have in their
doctors.

Education and training

The heritage of professional training within the primary care sector both at pre-
registration and post-registration levels, continuing professional development
and post-graduation education, has been *uniprofessional*.

*   Doctors have studied clinical medicine, clinical practice and the practice of
    being an *expert generalist*.
*   Nurses have studied the practice of nursing, the nursing process, nurse
    management and the specialist branches of nursing such as health visiting,

occupational health nursing and cancer nursing. In recent times the development of nurse prescribing and nurse triage, nurse led practice and specialist outreach nursing has meant more opportunities for nurses. However, they still learn and develop within the nursing profession.

- Pharmacists study medicine's management, therapeutics and clinical pharmacy with other pharmacists as part of the development of the profession of pharmacy.
- Other practitioner groups similarly have a heritage of education and training within their own practitioner group.

The support for such professional development has been channelled through universities and the NHS via a range of funding streams, professional allowances (such as PGEA) and professional requirements (such as PREP). This approach has served to perpetuate uniprofessional paradigms, professional development, and concepts of professionalism. However, this has frequently been divisive, with nurses resenting the power, autonomy and resources which have flowed into continuing medical education; and GPs, as employers of nurses as well as their professional colleagues in primary care teams, sometimes resenting having to fund education of practice nurses out of their own income as well as covering their clinical work when they are away. Nurses and other members of the primary care team employed by community and specialist trusts have had access to education and training programmes through their employers and have not faced some of the difficulties of practice nurses, but nevertheless the programmes provided for them have been focused largely around clinical practice needs. The requirement for education and training to support career development beyond clinical practice, dealing with issues such as management responsibilities, organisational development, human resource management, planning, financial management, leadership and strategic change, has seldom been available to practitioners from any of the clinical disciplines.

The involvement of the pharmaceutical industry in funding education and training for clinical practitioners has been influential in facilitating the development of continuing professional development. Without the support of the industry only a small fraction of the current activity could continue, the quality of the programmes would decline and the coverage of the workforce would be much more limited. However, funding by the pharmaceutical industry forms part of its marketing strategy designed to promote the use of its products. Although the marketing may be low key and the education programmes supported are 'non-promotional' nevertheless, any industry funding has to be in the interest of its shareholders.

The interests of the shareholders are best served by increasing sales of the company's products and by improving the image of the company in the eyes of the prescriber and his or her team. Pharmaceutical companies inevitably have less interest in clinical conditions where they have no treatment available, such as many of the inherited diseases and other conditions with low prevalence, but high morbidity, e.g. motor neurone disease and multiple sclerosis. They will tend to favour programmes which look at issues of high prevalence, but relatively low morbidity where higher profits can be made. These are, however, areas where they will have to compete with other companies for market share and develop sophisticated marketing strategies if they are to succeed.

Current developments in education and training are challenging this heritage of uniprofessional, clinically focused development through the development of *personal development, or personal, learning plans* and the linkage of these to organisational development plans such as *practice professional development plans*. Linking these individual plans – which should apply to all the primary care workforce, clinical and non-clinical – to programmes supported and organised through PCTs, can help those organisations develop as learning organisations (*see* Chapter 4). In addition, PCTs are frequently facing recruitment and retention difficulties for many grades of staff, and a high quality programme of personal development opportunities will be an important tool for them to help develop, recruit and retain staff. Valuing continual professional development, so that practitioners see it as an activity which is • central to their purpose rather than one which has to take place in 'their own time' • has corporate commitment from the PCT • is relevant to their needs and • over which they have a considerable input into the content and delivery mode, would be beneficial. Currently half-day once a month release programmes such as TARGET in Doncaster are proving popular. Covering the clinical commitment by extending 'out-of-hours GP co-op' cover has been helpful.

As PCTs develop and mature and as they explore their new responsibilities (*see* Chapter 7), so the education and training programmes they commission will undoubtedly evolve to support them in adapting to these new responsibilities. Such programmes will focus on their developing responsibilities into areas such as the following.

1   *Quality.* Quality of care, quality of care organisation, quality of care management, quality of communications, quality of design and quality assurance.
2   *Genetics.* Looking at the anatomy of genetics, DNA, etc., the impact of genetics on individuals and their families, the system for caring for people with genetic needs, such as genetic networks and genetic counselling, and the ethical implications of genetic medicine. The continuing work of the Human Genetics Commission supported by the government's commitment to a green paper on genetics illustrates the importance of this relatively underexplored area for PCTs. The implications of reports such as 'Whose hands on your genes?'[4] and 'Inside information'[5] deserve examination.
3   *Social exclusion.* Focusing programmes on areas of particular concern to the community such as the elderly and mentally infirm, substance abuse, adolescent behaviour, teenage pregnancy and homelessness so that the primary care workforce understands not just the disease management requirements

of these groups, but how improving their health can improve the health of the community.

4   *Welfare.* Exploring with the workforce how disease management and health improvement activities can link with voluntary sector and social care programmes to help reduce the risk that environmental problems such as poverty, unemployment, deprivation and ignorance will cascade through the generations and become just as much an inherited or genetic problem as those caused by abnormal DNA, such as muscular dystrophy or cystic fibrosis.

5   *Community development.* The primary care workforce are intimately involved with all aspects of their local communities. Understanding and supporting community development initiatives, such as youth work, housing action programmes, recreation and sporting activities, etc. and seeing how this work is contributing to the health of the community and the individuals who make it up, will be an important element in helping the workforce see their role in the context of broader definitions of health need – beyond the absence of disease and the prevention of disease, and towards personal fulfilment, achievement and active participation in, and giving to, the local community.

6   *Membership.* If the PCT is to become an organisation whose policies and functions are driven by the views and needs of the individuals making up its local communities, i.e. its members, then the opportunities for education and training that the organisation provides its workforce must also be extended to the rest of its membership. Individuals must be helped to address their own health needs to appreciate their own responsibility for their own inheritance, health and lifestyle and to understand the diseases that they suffer from. Helping them become 'expert patients' so that they can use the primary care professional workforce appropriately will help the PCT to bridge the divide between its workforce and its broader membership.

The primary care workforce forms, of course, an important section of the membership of the PCT. It is they who translate the policies and responsibilities of the trust board into day-to-day reality. It is they who need to appreciate and understand why the organisation and its culture are evolving:

•   from being a professionally dominated, patronising and paternalistic provider of disease management services
•   towards becoming a health maintaining and promoting organisation, driven by the needs of the individuals making up the local community and offered to that community as a professional and supportive advice, information and treatment service.

If we now look at the education and training implications of the responsibilities PCTs will have in Choice First and the Feel Good Factor then we can begin to appreciate how the use of education and training programmes by PCTs as 'change management agents' may develop.

Choice First

In this future we can see that there has been a coming together of the disparate training programmes which different practitioner groups have historically followed. Everyone starts off on a common course and gradually develops their particular specialism and expertise. Experienced practitioners had been offered 'grandfather' arrangements, but the workforce is now largely made up of people who have completed basic generic training and are working towards additional qualifications and modules. Once they have completed enough modules they are 'practitioner' trained and able to work in the treatment clinic seeing members face to face, but still working to protocols. Care managers must complete their own research programme, participate in a stringent supervised practice programme and write up a number of complex cases to a satisfactory standard. Each centre only employs a few care managers who are responsible for managing members with complex health problems. They have become recognised as 'expert generalists' comparable to the expert specialists working in referral centres. There are a few staff members in the treatment clinic who choose to specialise in *T&T* (triage and trauma) and they are able to go out to local accidents to provide emergency services. In addition, treatment clinics will be visited by specialists such as skin specialists, medicines advice specialists and psychotherapists.

We can see that in this *future* continuing development of the workforce is an essential core feature of the organisation's function, through:

- helping the workforce understand the responsibilities of the organisation in terms of organisational development, investment and capitalisation, workforce development, quality assurance and supervision by the National Standards Authority
- communication with, learning with and listening to its membership
- cost-effective care, personal investment accounts and understanding how the organisation is funded.

These issues, allied to the modular personal development programme, tailored for each individual, mean that the organisation is not only dealing with its recruitment and retention of staff priorities, but also ensuring that it is fit to meet its responsibilities.

The Feel Good Factor

This is a much smaller, more locally focused organisation than Choice First. Although its policies and ethos are established by its management committee, it is centrally regulated and performance is managed very rigorously. The emphasis is on ensuring a healthy environment for people to live and work in.

Each of the teams will have a senior practitioner. All team members have the same basic training up to NVQ level four, covering biological science, welfare law and community development. People have the option to take further training in specialist areas and to progress into either complex pathology managers (analogous to GPs and primary care physicians who transferred into the Bureau when it was formed) while others move into management areas or develop their expertise in audit, risk management and education so as to become practice standards directors (PSDs).

In this future the education and training programmes which the Bureau provides must primarily focus on developing the care teams. The programme will look at clinical competence and ensure that clinical practice is in line with central advice, but will be much more focused on team cohesion and effectiveness. Team roles, monitoring of team performance and the quality of care as perceived by individual patients, leadership and support, accessibility and feedback, care and health promotion will all be elements of team performance which team members will need to explore and be held to account for as part of the Bureau's management of team performance.

The workforce will be trained to encourage individual responsibility for health, improving and encouraging healthy lifestyles, risk avoidance and harm minimisation. Helping individuals understand and make informed choices about their lifestyle, their inheritance and their social responsibilities will require practitioners to develop further their empathetic and counselling skills and they will also need to understand and appreciate the importance of community spirit, community involvement and community support if their team performance is to be maximised.

The workforce will need to understand the role of the PSD and the place of quality assurance in maximising their individual and team effectiveness.

The Bureau's clinical teams are its operational arms. They are employed by the Bureau and have to understand and appreciate its functions, its policies, its governing arrangements and its priorities. Understanding what is the responsibility of the Bureau, and what is not, must be at the finger tips of every team member and therefore must form part of the education and training programmes. Realising that the Bureau's funding comes from central taxation and is contributed to by every individual, but that the funding is limited and focused on improving health and helping individuals take responsibility for their own lives, will be much more a feature of the Bureau's education programme than it is of PCTs.

Relationships

The second set of levers, or tools, which PCTs have at their disposal for support in addressing their new responsibilities are the relationship levers through which the trust's board and staff relate to other stakeholders within the local primary care sector and the wider welfare environment and community. The relationships with external stakeholders – such as those with local specialist services – also warrant consideration.

The background of organisations *within* the primary care sector has been of autonomous practices and small businesses, administered through national contractual frameworks, through quangos such as LHAs, executive committees, FHSAs etc. PCTs will need to deliver care across their range of responsibilities, through close working with the existing workforce and will wish to support them in meeting the challenges of their roles and responsibilities as these evolve and change. The needs of local communities will, to some extent, vary across the country and certainly PCT boards will wish to interpret policy and central direction within a local context so that they deliver their responsibilities in the light of current service abilities, existing relationships and local resources. To this end they are likely to wish to discuss with practices, businesses, voluntary sector and local authority departments the extent to which they can contribute towards the PCT's objectives and help the organisation discharge its responsi-bilities. The heritage of national contracts and administration may be insuf-ficiently flexible to allow PCTs to effectively discharge their responsibilities and they can therefore be expected to wish to promote more flexible and more locally sensitive arrangements to govern their working relationships.

Early experiments towards such flexibilities formed part of the experience under fundholding, total purchasing and locality commissioning in the 1990s and are being further developed through personal medical services/personal dental services/local pharmaceutical services pilots. These seek to interpret and address local priorities through developing new ways of working and new con-tractual relationships between PCTs and local provider organisations. Addressing the needs of particular community groups such as refugees and the homeless; encouraging alternative career options such as salaried partners or nurse directed practices; encouraging practices to address particular local issues beyond their national contractual obligations such as drug and alcohol services, specialist dermatology or education roles; exploring e-prescribing and medicines manage-ment programmes; developing new NHS dental services with salaried practitioners; offering improved access arrangements and triage through walk-in centres and out-of-hours co-operatives are all current developments which seek to link PCTs to service flexibility and improvement at a local level. While PCTs will learn much about local contracting through these pilots dealing with particular local cir-cumstances, they will also wish to discuss with every primary care practitioner how they can contribute to the priorities of the PCT. Until dialogue between the PCT and its constituents is backed by the power of resource allocation, account-ability relationships and an appreciation of the power and responsibilities of each party, such discussions are likely to be exploratory and supportive rather than constructive, productive and challenging. The variation in the way practitioners have delivered services, the resources they have consumed and the quality of their management and clinical practice have previously defied close examination and measurement. PCTs will need to agree with the providers how these issues are to be managed and will require considerable expertise to do this sensitively and constructively. It is not yet clear where such expertise and understanding is to come from and how it is to develop, but the success of PCTs in discharging their responsibilities will be heavily dependent upon it.

Such partnerships with local providers, based as they have to be on mutual respect and trust, agreement about the roles and responsibilities of each party, the resources to be committed to agreed programmes of work and the monitoring arrangements of the partnership, will all be important. In addition, arrangements with other PCTs around joint commissioning to meet their shared objectives, e.g. specialist services, transport, out-of-hours care, etc., will be required and may be formalised through forms of service level agreement. Relationships with local authority departments, perhaps involving joint appointments, joint membership of each other's committees and board, shared policies, planning cycles and approaches and jointly managed projects will be very much in the interests of the PCTs as they move into their community development responsibilities.

Working relationships with voluntary sector organisations will also need to evolve. Administrative support and project funding should never seek to stifle the lifeblood of the voluntary sector which is its responsiveness to local circumstance and to the gaps which exist in statutory care provision. The voluntary sector is often a vital indicator, or lightening conductor, serving to illustrate the areas where PCTs will need to focus their energies. The PCTs will need to learn from local voluntary sector organisations as well as support them; they will need to involve them in their planning processes, policy-making forums and commissioning frameworks, but without seeking to neuter them. PCTs and voluntary sector organisations will also need to appreciate that there is frequently a bias involved in their relationship. Voluntary organisations will not have an overview of all the issues surrounding their area of interest – consider the Cystic Fibrosis Trust, the Red Cross or the WRVS – and they will not be unbiased in their views or appreciate or give weight to the issues outside their area of interest, for example over issues of child protection, cancer treatment or prescribing. Nevertheless, involving the voluntary sector and through them the interest groups they serve can be vital in engaging with patient groups such as The British Diabetic Association, Cystic Fibrosis Trust and Multiple Sclerosis Society who can contribute so much to the management of their own disease.

Box 8.2:   Case study

At the Derbyshire Dales and South Derbyshire PCG Health Improvement Program Conference in 2000 it became apparent that the local authorities planned to allow the building of an additional 5000 houses in the area, which would have implications for local health services. Joint working between the PCG and the local authority housing and planning departments helped them understand the implications of the myriad of small developments which made up these plans for community development over the next

10 years, and led to the PCT board agreeing short, medium and longer term plans to address the 10 000–15 000 expected population growth. Local services were already full to capacity with average GP list sizes of over 2000, little or no availability of local NHS dentistry, some difficulty in recruiting and retaining particular nursing groups, as well as GPs, and a lack of capacity in the buildings and infrastructure of primary care to meet the needs of the increase in population.

Already in 2001 the majority of general practices in the area had closed their books and capped their lists, so that patients were having difficulty in finding a new doctor and patient choice was being constrained. Many patients were being forced to pay for private dentistry while those unable to pay were often inappropriately consulting general medical practitioners about dental problems. The overstretched community dental service was unable to expand its capacity.

Planning between the PCG and local primary care providers meant that the short term solution was the development of a PMS project with a local practice where they would employ an additional salaried PMS partner, expand their surgery capacity by opening their branch surgery for extra hours, and expand their ancillary and nursing teams to cope with an additional 1500 patients over the following two years. PMS arrangements meant that this expansion in capacity could be 'front-loaded' to ensure that the practice list remained open and that the additional provision could be planned and developed in a co-ordinated way. It should be appreciated that the national GMS approach through establishing a new practice with initial practice allowances, etc., while an option, was not considered sufficiently flexible for the local phased development programme.

The next phase is planned to be the establishment of a PMS project linking several other local practices, with shared additional practitioner resources to deal with the increasing population.

In the longer run it is anticipated that a new practice will be formed on a site which currently houses community services, the GPs' out-of-hours co-operative, and an old redundant ambulance station. This development may not be needed for 3–5 years, but the early identification and planning between the local authority and the PCG means that all parties can design the primary care service more proactively than in the past.

PCTs have inherited responsibility for a more formal framework of relationships with specialist, secondary care, providers. The SAFF (service and financial framework) is the agreement between the specialist trusts and health authorities (now with PCTs) about who will do what for whom, how much it will cost and what developments and changes will be encouraged. Rather than the contractual relationships which characterised the internal market during the 1990s, the SAFF process is meant to develop a more flexible partnership ethos among the local health service family. Thus far the experience of SAFF and the influence primary care has had over the process has been disappointing. The specialist provider's 'wish list', national imperatives and unavoidable cost pressures, have meant little progress on reconfiguring care pathways, transferring resources to support transferring care, developing intermediate services or quality assurance. PCTs will need to consider how the SAFF process can evolve to include all the budgets involved (including GMS, prescribing, management costs and HCHS) and become an instrument for modernising health service delivery rather than a closed shop agreement fixing financial baselines.

What can the two 'futures' tell us about the way relationships between the elements making up the primary care sector might develop over the next few years?

Choice First

First Call is part of Choice First and is linked to a number of local *first stop* treatment clinics. In addition there are a number of satellite clinics or *first aid* centres linked to Choice First. It is important to remember that all the staff working in, or in association with, Choice First are employed by it. In addition, they are encouraged to become shareholders in it, i.e. members of it, and just as individual citizens become members of Choice First and commit their individual savings account to the organisation, so the staff commit their careers and career development. This relationship between the elements of Choice First ensure its cohesion and help it address its responsibilities, including sensitivity to its members' views and the requirement for quality assurance and evidence based practice. The contractual relationships with specialist care providers has meant transfer of resource and responsibility into Choice First and, in response to major technological innovation, considerable consolidation of specialist care.

The Feel Good Factor

The relationship between the care providing primary care teams in this future and the Bureau and its management committee is one of much more performance management by the Bureau than is the case between PCTs and local practices. While it is likely that many of the primary care team members will be directly employed by the Bureau, it is also likely that the health improving and the community spirit focused ethos of the Bureau will mean that a considerable proportion of team members will be part-time, voluntary workers and employed by other agencies, such as education or local private sector employers. The focus on managing team performance as a *team* will make the responsibility for managing the relationships between employed team members and other team members the responsibility of the team rather than of the Bureau itself.

Because the Bureau sees itself very much as part of the local community it can be expected that it will have close and well defined working relationships with other community organisations, such as the voluntary groups, local authority and private organisations.

Resources transferred from hospital to the community have helped develop the capacity, within the community, for additional locally based care, supported by specialist providers rather than dependent on them.

Resource allocation

The third area of leverage that the PCTs will need to develop to improve the quality of care their communities receive and to deliver on their full range of responsibilities as they develop will involve their use of resources. In the past the primary care sector was funded from a variety of funding streams. Historically there have been two main funding streams allocated by Parliament to resource the NHS.

1   The first, known as the HCHS budget (Hospital and Community Health Services budget), has been used to pay for specialist services such as those provided by NHS hospitals and also those provided by community trusts such as district nursing, health visiting, etc. HCHS funds also provide for specialist mental health services and their community teams, learning disability services, including community homes and community paediatric services, including child protection and child and adolescence psychiatry.

2   The second funding stream from Parliament, the GMS budget (General Medical Services budget), has resourced the services provided by independent contractors, such as GPs, community pharmacy, community dentistry and community optician services. The greater proportion of these budgets has been used to pay for general medical practice where it has funded practice nurses, management and ancillary staff, premises and IT infrastructure and GP incomes. It should be appreciated that as independent contractors GPs, dentists, pharmacists etc. remain self-employed and use all the GMS resource allocated to their practice to pay for the infrastructure, before living off the remaining or residual funds as their income. This obviously introduces an incentive for GPs to underinvest in their practice so as to maximise their income and, given that their funding allocation is largely based on capitation and history rather than the identified needs of their registered list, there is little flexibility for resources to be redistributed between practices.

An increasingly large proportion of the resources consumed within the primary care sector is involved with the supply of medicines through prescribing and dispensing arrangements. Although in most cases these do not directly affect most GPs' incomes, they do affect pharmacists' incomes and GPs, where they act as dispensing doctors, are also affected. Thus far there has been little incentive for prescribers and dispensers to address issues such as the cost-effectiveness of their prescribing performance, but the consequences of their prescribing do affect all the other budgets, e.g. GMS and HCHS. PCTs have to manage all the funds at their disposal and achieve financial balance, which means that any overspend on prescribing has to be balanced by an underspend elsewhere and this has to be achieved each year, rather than carried forward or balanced by carrying forward underspends from previous years. This rigid financial framework for PCTs also includes the requirement for them to manage the majority of the HCHS budget through commissioning specialist services, i.e. the majority of hospital services.

Pressures for increased emergency admissions or outpatient appointments or problems with waiting list management will have to be considered by PCT boards alongside pressures in prescribing or GMS budgets.

The freedom to vire resources between the different budgets for which PCTs are responsible has been severely limited throughout the history of the NHS. Although some virement was permitted through the fundholding scheme and within tightly regulated arrangements by health authorities, this never included the freedom to move money out of the GMS budget into the HCHS budget.

PCTs are new, largely autonomous, organisations which will inevitably seek the freedom to organise and resource the care for their local populations, without the rigid constraints of history. The freedom to provide care where technology and patient choice dictates and to move the resources from hospital to community or vice versa to support that care will be essential. In addition, the freedom to vire resources to support different therapeutic options will be required. While drug treatment may be appropriate in some cases, physiotherapy, occupational therapy, hydrotherapy, massage, homeopathic treatment, acupuncture or psychotherapy may be appropriate alternatives. PCTs will need to be able to offer the local community access to this range of alternative treatments and to resource them in the same way as drugs are resourced. This may mean challenging prescribing behaviour and the marketing and promotional activities of the pharmaceutical industry and vireing resources from prescribing to support other alternative therapies. PCTs will have to reflect that their responsibilities extend beyond the purely medical paradigms of health and disease into improving health and preventing disease, and as such will need to identify and focus resources to address these responsibilities.

As time moves on new technology permits change in the way care is delivered – the use of mobile phones, video cameras and alarm buzzers has had impact over the last decade, and we can predict further technological innovation and changing care provision in future years. Budgetary inflexibility makes the introduction of such new technologies difficult unless special central resource is provided, e.g. for IM&T development. PCTs will need to plan for such innovations and have the freedom to vire resources between different budget heads to meet technological change as well as local circumstance.

The development of care trusts and teaching trusts means that PCTs may also be considering social care budgets and pre-registration education budgets, as part of their resource, while all PCTs will have educational responsibilities as part of their change management and service development programmes. Some may choose to focus on teaching in partnership with local universities to a greater extent. These teaching trusts are being established in areas where recruitment and retention of practitioners has been particularly difficult and are seen as a way of improving the standard of care that patients receive in those areas. PCTs will need to be able to vire resources to support this teaching focus which will inevitably have implications for primary care infrastructure, GMS budget, prescribing, etc.

PCTs which choose to become 'care trusts' and take on responsibilities for social care as well as healthcare will similarly need to be able to vire resources between social care budgets and healthcare budgets to develop flexible responses to the needs of their local community. Difficult issues, such as whether the client pays for his or her own care, have bedevilled partnership arrangements between health and social care in the past and will inevitably prove challenging for care trusts.

The Feel Good Factor

This is the centrally resourced future where the Healthy Living Bureau will seek to use its resources to promote health in a much more holistic and co-ordinated fashion than PCTs can currently envisage. The Bureau will use the resources at its disposal to promote health, foster personal responsibilities and community spirit; to promote healthier lifestyles and challenge 'deviant' behaviour. The shift away from specialist care in institutions and towards community provision will have facilitated and resourced this approach and the move away from a pharmaceutical definition of therapy towards a more holistic and broader definition of care will have allowed a redistribution of resource and virement of funds from a medical model approach to a paradigm of care based around community spirit, health improvement and community partnership. At the same time the Bureau will be centrally performance managed against national standards, will need to follow guidance and address national priorities. This remains a National Health Service, but not as it has been defined in the past.

The Bureau will have consigned traditional medical records to history. All team members will share a common record of care, which will be the patient's property. With so much care being provided at home by so many team members, effective co-ordination and communication have become vital – good care depends on that. The Bureau is held to account because the teams are performance managed on their effectiveness and investment to support team working is a key priority for the whole organisation.

Choice First

In this world there has been radical change to the funding streams through which healthcare is provided. The implementation of personal investment accounts has meant that the board of Choice First has to offer a range of products which attract members to invest their accounts with the organisation. This is analogous to the range of options available to members of health clubs and fitness centres in the early years of the twenty-first century and the range of membership opportunities open to those joining sports clubs. From the available resource provided by the members or other funders, such as local employers, insurance companies, financial institutions, shareholders and the voluntary sector, the board will decide how to provide care and meet its diverse responsibilities. The organisation has not only to balance its books, but also address the issues of investment while remaining a 'not for profit' organisation. As is clear from the description (listen to the audio files at www.radcliffe-oxford.com/challenge) the board is actively considering whether to end its not for profit status and become a private sector limited company. The requirement for investment is of a magnitude which it is difficult to sustain within the constraints of its public sector ethos and, if it is to remain at the leading edge of development, additional funds may be required and a kind of public–private partnership arrangement, as has developed in transport, specialist care and education, is being considered.

Choice First will use all the resources at its disposal to plan the care packages demanded by its members and required by the National Standards Authority. It will fund the infrastructure, such as education and training, workforce development and quality assurance programmes and vire resources between primary and secondary care or specialist and community based care to support service reconfiguration. The dramatic decrease in the use of institutional specialist care has released resources to develop high quality specialist care in the community, largely delivered through the First Call care programme approach. Direct employment of the vast majority of First Call staff has meant less difficulty vireing resources between budget heads and more flexibility over redesigning care packages, without affecting the take home pay of any group in the workforce.

Individual members are responsible for their own clinical records – all staff contribute to them, on line, at the time of consultation – and all staff have access to the complete record if the member agrees. The days of paper based records of medical care, nursing care, hospital care, pharmacy support and social care interventions have ended – it is just not safe for patients, staff or First Call, giving rise to too many lawsuits and too many hidden errors.

Sadly the ever larger and larger organisation has restricted choice and the government is becoming concerned about such restrictions. Referral to the Monopolies and Mergers Authority may act as a constraint acting against the economies of scale that large organisations offer.

Operational and planning tools

In order to develop the leverage in the three areas outlined above – change management through education and training, more dynamic relationships and resource allocation – the new corporate primary care organisations such as PCTs will need to use a range of operational tools. Further development of existing instruments, such as those used by health authorities, educationalists and private sector management and adapting them to use in the primary care sector has provided a useful starting point, but there is much more to be done. To move on from the heritage of general management with varying clinical involvement or engagement into a future where the motivated clinical workforce leads and directs primary care into a future which better addresses the needs of all individuals within the community, requires PCTs (and their peers in Scotland, Wales and Northern Ireland) to focus on:

- personal development of all those with responsibility for leadership and managing change in the PCT
- *general* management skills for clinicians with management responsibilities, and *clinical* management skills for general managers with clinical areas of responsibility: clinicians must be enabled to effectively direct and deliver change in clinical services, and reconfigure the care packages patients receive; managers who understand clinical perspectives can facilitate change through the application of management principles
- understanding the place of national initiatives such as NSFs, NICE guidance, the CHI remit, professional revalidation and reaccreditation, performance management through SHAs, etc.

Before exploring each of these in a little more detail it is worth reflecting that PCTs will develop their own ways of addressing these issues and interpret their responsibilities in the light of local circumstances. Initiatives such as whole PCT Personal Medical Services projects, PCT half-day closure education programmes, piloting development in one 'exemplar' practice, promoting service reconfiguration in particular areas as in 'exemplars', e.g. intermediate care services or near patient anticoagulation services – these and others might be appropriate in different localities. Lessons will need to be learned from the successes and failures of these initiatives so that all PCTs can benefit from the experience of others, and adapt that experience to their local circumstances.

One of the areas where primary care has historically been underdeveloped is in the use of planning tools. Thus far the primary care sector has essentially been reactive – general practice has responded to what comes through the door and community pharmacy to the behaviour and habits of prescribers and customers. Primary care and community nursing have responded to acute sector and general practice behaviour and indeed it is fair to say that none of the sub-units of the primary care sector have had sufficient autonomy and freedom to manoeuvre, to be able to effectively plan development coherently. PCTs will need to introduce a culture of planning in order to ensure the safety of care and resources and deliver change in a way that has the confidence of the stakeholders. Primary care practitioners will need help to understand planning processes, cycles, tools and constraints and will bring a somewhat jaundiced view with them. In becoming a more planned sector of care there is a risk that the innovation, flexibility, sensitivity to patients' individual and personal requirements and the independence of the independent contractor organisations will be lost and replaced by a planned care system providing worse care. Practitioners will need to be convinced by the PCT that there is no need to 'throw the baby out with the bath water' – that it is perfectly possible to retain the good aspects of the sector's heritage while introducing the advantages of planning. The engagement of clinicians and other staff in the primary care sector in the planning processes of the PCT will be essential if their jaundiced view, cynicism, etc. is to change. PCTs will need to go to considerable lengths to consult, learn from clinicians, interpret and build consensus, lead from behind as well as in front and be prepared to temper their zeal for change by respecting the need for it to be managed over a period of time so as not to destabilise current service provisions.

The use of tools such as scenario planning,[6] which was used to develop the *Tomorrow's World* primary care futures (Choice First and the Feel Good Factor), is one approach that PCTs could look at. It involves synthesising the view of stakeholders and, through a formal process, developing consensus as to what the stakeholders are trying to achieve and supports decision making about how to prepare and plan for those achievements. The techniques have been widely used in the private sector, e.g. by Shell to plan for their future following oil price rises of the 1970s, by the public sector such as the NHS and by nation states such as South Africa in planning for its future in the post-apartheid world. The common theme has been using the technique to build consensus among stakeholders before deciding on alternative options and helping decision makers make better decisions by engaging all stakeholders in the process, i.e. the thesis is that *better decisions are made if the process for making them is better*. There are of course alternatives – the use of focus groups and other similar tools and qualitative research methods such as the use of questionnaires, interviews, feedback reports, observations and facilitated discussions, may all play a part in helping PCTs to plan ahead.

Leadership

Current plans by the modernisation agency for leadership programmes in primary care, focusing initially on PCT chairs, chief executives and the chairs of professional executive committees (PECs), offer a welcome if long delayed recognition that leadership is an important function in the primary care sector. Past leadership programmes for health authority and NHS trust directors and clinicians have meant a considerable investment in developing the leadership capacity of the health service and some individuals who have gone through these programmes will no doubt apply their experience in PCTs. Nevertheless, the failure to offer leadership and personal development to individuals and teams facing major change and challenges in the primary care sector has meant that the development of a *primary care led health service* through the late 1980s and 1990s has been constrained by its lack of capacity and its lack of any kind of leadership and representative culture.

There are many different definitions and types of leadership – it is probably best looked at as a quality, with various different dimensions, rather than as a function or task. The style of leadership and the functions of leadership within any PCT will inevitably need to be sensitive to local circumstance and change with time. However, individuals facing responsibilities within PCTs and the broader sector will be much better equipped to meet their responsibilities and the challenges involved if they understand and are confident with different leadership styles and approaches, if they can develop insight into their own preferred approaches and appreciate the requirements of the individuals, teams and organisations with which they work. Once again, reflecting back to Chapter 4 may help appreciate some of the dimensions and functions which leadership in PCTs will need to address.

Clinical management

Perhaps one of the most powerful, but underdeveloped, tools to provide leverage over the whole healthcare system that PCTs have at their disposal is provided by their clinicians. These individuals have a range of professional backgrounds and have had operational responsibilities for all the issues that PCT boards are facing.

- Through their direct provider functions they can appreciate the scale and extent of pathology within the local community.
- They will know the strengths and opportunities for further development as well as areas of relative weakness in the local pattern of care.
- As employers and managers of their businesses they will understand the local labour market and the requirements for workforce developments.
- As owners and capitalisers of their businesses they will be aware of the capital and financial circumstances facing the PCT.
- As referrers to, and colleagues of, clinicians throughout the rest of the healthcare system they will be aware of the history and circumstances which affect the quality of care their patients receive beyond the consulting rooms.

Empowering clinicians to take responsibility for managing change within the PCT and beyond must not risk damaging the capacity of the PCT to provide its clinical services – general practitioners have to remain expert generalist clinicians, but will need to adapt their roles so that they are less diverted to meeting the demands of the worried well, rather than the requirements of those with greatest health needs. There is currently a great danger that the demand led primary care practitioner workforce of GPs, nurses, pharmacists, etc. may be forced to behave like hamsters in a wheel – running faster and faster, but never moving anywhere, overburdened by process so that they can never look at outcome. Developing clinicians with management and planning skills so that they can act as clinical leaders and clinical managers will be an essential tool for PCTs in their task of delivering on their responsibilities for providing care, commissioning care and working in partnership as well as understanding the health needs of their communities.[7]

At the same time managers developing their careers in the primary care sector will need to adapt their general management skills and experience to the culture of the primary care sector. Financial management, human resource management, estate management, corporate affairs, planning, etc. will all need to be adapted and implemented in ways which are sensitive to the primary care sector's heritage in order to manage the performance of independent contractors in the same way that health authorities have negotiated and managed processes such as the SAFF process with acute trusts or use public health physicians as clinical change agents, conducting speciality reviews and negotiating clinical change. Appreciating the advantages of the flexible, autonomous, independent nature of primary care small businesses, appreciating the power which clinicians wield through their referral and prescribing responsibilities and understanding how important is the trust, respect and faith which individuals have in their primary care practitioners, will be essential for managers in PCTs. They need to work in partnership with clinicians within their organisation, which means:

- trusting and respecting each other
- agreeing what needs to be done, how to do it and how to ensure that lessons are learnt along the way, plans are revisited and changing circumstances are taken into account.

In some acute trusts the experience of clinical directors and general managers can provide lessons for PCTs in how to effectively manage change and work together, in others the lessons might be how not to do it – nevertheless the lessons can be valuable.

Any new contractual arrangements for clinicians or general managers will have to reflect their changing responsibilities. The extent to which current discussions about a new contract for GPs[8] and other discussions for other groups reflect their changing responsibilities and support the development of appropriate relationships will be another criterion for judging the quality of the contractual frameworks.

Central initiatives

PCTs have to appreciate that in a NHS, funded nationally and accountable to Parliament, there will inevitably be national priorities which PCTs will need to deliver on. In addition, there will be common issues among all PCTs which will be better explored and directed nationally, so that energies are not wasted by reinventing wheels at local level. Perhaps the guide should be that work is only undertaken at PCT level if it can only be done there and that work is only undertaken nationally or at SHA level if it adds value to PCT level work.

Examples of national work include national service frameworks[9] and these are useful tools for PCTs to use to provide leverage for change in service planning and development in their localities. Each of the NSFs has provided a framework which looks beyond the traditional disease management and medical model approach to a national issue. Examples such as coronary heart disease, mental health and services for the elderly[9] look at the need for a planned delivery of healthcare, the factors influencing disease management and health improvement and the changes that are going on in society that contribute to the health needs and provide a programme for improving services at local levels. Using the NSF to focus PCTs' energies makes a lot of sense, although requiring every PCT to produce local guidelines on the management of key areas in mental health has meant a great deal of reinventing wheels around the country.

The process of nationally assessing the clinical and cost effectiveness of treatment is through NICE[10] which has been important, although somewhat controversial. Inevitably there are powerful voices who see their power to proffer or use treatments being curtailed and who resent and criticise the way that NICE has developed. PCTs would do well to remember that the purpose of NICE is to ensure the availability of effective treatment to the whole population and that NICE is producing guidance for PCTs and local clinicians over issues which would otherwise consume large amounts of energy in every local PCT. Although the processes and procedures may need to evolve and change, the responsibility to assess clinical and cost-effectiveness and ensure that patients receive effective treatment which is value for money will not go away.

Quality assurance is an essential part of ensuring that the users of the service have confidence in it. Patients need to trust their doctors and the community needs to have confidence in their hospitals and in the organisations which run the health service. The CHI, by visiting, inspecting and reporting on the quality of care provided by all NHS practitioners, can provide that objective view about the quality of care provided and ensure that the individual and community's trust and confidence in the service is not misplaced. The further development of CHI to assume responsibility for aspects of the Audit Commission's responsibilities (becoming CHIA), announced recently, also demonstrates how important holistic quality assurance is to the development of *high trust* relationships between PCTs and the rest of the health service. PCTs will also need to develop their own quality assurance mechanisms to back up the CHIA process so that they are prepared for their visits and to ensure that the trust patients put in them is not misplaced. The primary care history of flexible, innovative and independent practice is no guarantee of high quality, and systems will need to be put in place by PCTs to drive up the quality of care which patients receive. The clinical governance responsibility of PCT chief executives, and that of the clinical governance leads within each PCT, is important because it brings together responsibility across all the quality assurance areas, e.g.:

- risk management
- education and training
- compliance
- audit and review.

This will be required to underpin the quality improvement programme within the PCT.

Choice First

The use of the toolkit discussed above has enabled Choice First to develop rapidly. There remains a strong quality assurance ethic in the organisation which is responsive to the requirements of the National Standards Authority. It is important that the organisation is accredited and accountable to its funders – be they individuals through their PIAs or insurance companies, employers or shareholders.

The Feel Good Factor

This remains at heart a public service organisation, regularly reviewed by Off Health – formed by the merger of the functions of the Audit Commission and the Health Ombudsmen. It is also important to this future that the Practice Standards Director (PSD) keeps the teams 'up to scratch' with their clinical practice, ensuring that the care they provide is in line with the evidence and in ways which are both clinically and cost effective. This is important for the Bureau as a way of maintaining the confidence of the community. The Bureau does have the freedom to use alternative therapies such as *rest and recuperation, massage and homeopathy* but will, no doubt, need to convince Offhealth that provision of these is in line with its responsibility to provide effective, high quality care.

References

1 Department of Health (1999) *Supporting Doctors, Protecting Patients*. DoH, London.
2 Department of Health (2001) *Assuring the Quality of Medical Practice*. DoH, London.
3 Department of Health (2001) *Harold Shipman's Clinical Practice 1974–1998*. DoH, London.
4 *Whose Hands on Your Genes?* (2001) www.hgc.gov.uk
5 *Inside Information* (2002) www.hgc.gov.uk

6 IDON (1997) IDON Scenario Thinking. IDON Ltd. www.idongroup.com

7 Department of Health (1997) *The New NHS: modern, dependable*. DoH White Paper, London.

8 GMC/NHS Confederation (2002) *The New GMS Contract*. GMC, London.

9 Department of Health (2001) *National Service Framework – Older People*. DoH, London.

10 www.nice.org.uk

CHAPTER 9

Emerging issues

As the community revolution of the twenty-first century unfolds following the industrial and social revolutions of previous centuries, so definitions of professionalism, personal responsibility and care provision are all being questioned.

This chapter will consider a number of issues that PCTs are currently struggling with, or which are moving into the foreground. These are all issues which will mould the agenda of PCTs over the next few years and which have been addressed in the Feel Good Factor and Choice First futures (available at www.radcliffe-oxford.com/challenge). While some relevant and related issues, such as genetic medicine and skill substitution, have been considered in previous chapters, there remain a number of other areas that need further consideration. It is also worth reiterating that while new issues are emerging and new responsibilities are developing, unless there is an equivalent transfer of responsibilities out of the primary care sector, there will be an ever increasing risk of overloading and overstraining the capacity of the sector.

In this chapter we will consider new aspects of professionalism.

- We will consider professional roles, responsibilities and relationships as well as professional values and behaviour patterns and the structures that have underpinned them in the past and which are now adapting for the future.
- We will then look at some aspects of how the pattern of care patients receive is being reconfigured in the light of organisational, social and technological change, before considering the issue of the PCT as a disease management or health improvement organisation.
- We will consider the PCT as a membership organisation driven by the needs and aspirations of the individuals making up the local community.
- The issues raised by skill substitution, including the new professional roles that we dealt with earlier and also the issues of access to care, career development and clinical management will be considered further.
- Finally we need to look at the emerging technologies and how well they will impact on the care provided in the sector. This must consider electronic patient records, confidentiality through iris screening or pin numbers, distributed care of the elderly and vulnerable by remote supervision, access to laboratory tests and results online or via text messaging, and the issue of sharing the capacity and skills of the primary care workforce in the area.

This chapter then looks at the current themes emerging for PCTs and will do so against the backdrop of the *Tomorrow's World* futures, which must act as the perspective to these discussions. If we consider these futures to be 10 to 15 years ahead, then this chapter looks at steps towards these futures. Inevitably the themes discussed will have greater relevance to some PCTs because of their particular situation, and less relevance to others which may be facing other pressures. These themes then will need to be interpreted locally and, as has been discussed elsewhere in this book, will be influenced by all the forces acting on the PCT, such as its economic position, size, local relationships between providers of care, and the structure and cultural values of the local population.

Professionalism

The elements, which make up the heritage of professional behaviour in the primary care sector, are having to evolve and change.

Box 9.1: Professionalism

- Keyholder for a defined body of knowledge.
- Registered as qualified to practise.
- Self-regulation.
- Ethical standards.
- Code of conduct.

Box 9.1 summarises the heritage of professionalism. This heritage has developed from Victorian and Edwardian legacies.

- *Respect and deference.* The social order before the Second World War marked out the *professional* as coming from a different social group from the rest of the community that he or she worked within. His or her professional status was respected and judgement trusted; the professional's right of ownership of a defined body of knowledge was acknowledged.
- *Acceptance* that the community should not seek to control the professions, but should allow them sufficient autonomy so that their members could act for individual citizens, and be trusted by those citizens to be independent of state control.
- The *maintenance* and upholding of a set of *ethical* standards and the *code of conduct* by professional councils such as the GMC and UKCC illustrated this, and their power to remove members from their register remains an important element in maintaining that power.

Society at the beginning of the twenty-first century has moved on, and its respect and deference to professionals and its attitude to their autonomy has changed.

This change has affected all professions including the clergy, teachers, lawyers and accountants as well as the caring professions such as medicine and nursing. The characteristics of professionalism have been slowly evolving in response to such changes in society and PCTs will need to reflect on them.

Is it still relevant to be a 'keyholder for a defined body of knowledge' in a world of universal access to information via the Internet? The role may now be better defined as an 'interpreter of information' and as an adviser about the appropriateness of the information. Recent concerns of parents about vaccination issues, be it whooping cough or MMR, illustrate the extent to which they distrust advice from politicians and increasingly from their professional advisers, and wish to make up their own minds. If they are to retain confidence in the members of the caring professions, then they will only do so if they believe that those professionals are interpreting the evidence and advising them what is best for them – and their children – in the light of all circumstances, rather than: (i) telling them what to do; (ii) acting as the agent of the community or government; or (iii) denying them access to evidence, knowledge and information.

Box 9.2:   Hierarchy of control

- Data.
- Information.
- Knowledge.
- Wisdom.

Box 9.2 can be used to examine this issue. Whereas individual citizens may have access to the *data* about immunisation, i.e. the percentage population coverage needed to prevent outbreaks, the current immunisation rate, its cost and availability, information about its effectiveness, contraindications, side effects, recommended timing and how to access the scheme. On the basis of this data and *information* they will face pressure to take control, make decisions and act in the interests of their children. However, they recognise that they may lack an appreciation and understanding of the broader issues surrounding these decisions about immunisation – such as the risks of the disease that they are deciding to prevent by immunisation and its complications, the natural history of epidemics, viral genetic drift and the nature of viral infection with their long-term implications and possible effects on somatic cell genetics. They will therefore look to their professional advisers to support them in making their decisions by translating the information at their disposal into *knowledge*, by putting that information in the context of their own circumstances. *Wisdom* implies the synthesis of data, information and knowledge, reflection on them and then the application of them in a way which balances all the perspectives involved. It may be too much to expect that the caring professions can be seen as supporting citizens in making wise choices and decisions about their healthcare, but in the modern world it has to be steps towards this that move our concepts of professionalism into the modern world.

Other aspects of professionalism also need to be reviewed in the light of the way that society is evolving. Being registered as qualified to practise was important in a world where unqualified practitioners were able to practise and harm citizens with only limited risk of exposure. In a world of instant media attention and universal access to information the maintenance of a register of those 'qualified to practise' may seem out of date. Nevertheless, ensuring that all healthcare practitioners are *fit to practise* is vital. If the public is to have confidence in the practitioners then the product has to be quality assured. This quality assurance cannot be only at the time of qualification, but has to be continuous throughout practitioners' careers. In a world where quality assurance leads to phone calls and questionnaires from the garage after your car is serviced, league tables, OFSTED inspection of schools and television programmes, e.g. Watchdog, focusing on quality of service, the caring professions cannot remain isolationists.

Self-regulation then remains an important issue. If individual citizens are to retain confidence in the caring professions, then they must be convinced that professions have sufficient autonomy to be able to challenge the government's and community's perspective, and be immune to interference for 'political' reasons. Self-regulation should be about ensuring the confidence of those putting their faith and trust in the profession rather than about promoting the status and independence of the profession. To maintain and promote that confidence it would seem sensible that the regulatory machinery and processes are open to public scrutiny and involve independent representatives of the community – and lay members – who can ensure appropriate openness.

The ethical standards and codes of conduct which underpin professional behaviour remain as relevant as ever to concepts of professionalism. Nevertheless they need to mature with society so that they reflect the dilemmas and concerns of that society as it changes. The new ethical problems raised by globalisation, the post-family society and genetic medicine must inform the codes of conduct and ethical framework if they are to remain as relevant and vibrant parts of the healthcare systems.

If these are some of the *generic* issues which affect professional behaviour in the early years of PCTs then there are some specific issues which the professions involved in providing primary care need to consider. Table 9.1 summarises some of the issues for different professions and we shall consider them in a little more detail.

General practitioner

If we consider Choice First and the Feel Good Factor then we can see that the role of the general practitioner has altered radically in both. The underpinning

Table 9.1: Professional roles in PCTs

From	To
General Practitioner	
Expert generalist	Clinical care director
Registration	Membership
Gatekeeping	Enabling
Independence	Interdependence
Nurse	
Personal care	Health promotion
Nursing process	Care management
Reactive	Proactive
Pharmacist	
Dispenser	Medicines manager
Therapeutics adviser	Clinical pharmacist
Small shopkeeper	Managed care agent
External safety net	Team member

features of the professional role of the general practitioner in the last part of the twentieth century have included being an expert generalist.

This has defined the *body of knowledge* and areas of expertise of the general practitioner. That knowledge deals with disease which is generally prevalent or common in the community and at a level which supports the care for the generality of patients with those diseases during the majority of the time that they suffer from them. This requires the general practitioner to have expertise across all specialities, but to a depth which is less than that required of a specialist. The expertise is not just in the pathology, but also in the social and spiritual aspects of care which broaden the expert generalist function from being a pure physician role to a more holistic approach. Expert generalism implies interpreting pathology in the light of the personal circumstances of the patient and applying all the therapeutic options to the benefit of the patient. As the focus of the primary care sector moves from disease management to improving the health of the population, so the use of tools – such as NSFs – to focus attention on particular areas of care, will improve the overall quality of care provided by the expert generalist, but there is always the risk that the expertise of any general practitioner will not be balanced equally across all areas and all pathologies. Expert generalism implies a broad, but not particularly deep, knowledge across all areas, but increasingly, specialisation in particular areas, e.g. dermatology or gynaecology, is challenging expert generalism. The provision of the highest quality of care to every patient presenting to the general practitioner challenges the capacity of expert generalism, particularly given that the average consultation length is less than 10 minutes.

In future the role of the expert generalist[1] would seem to be to move in the direction of becoming a *clinical care director*.

Box 9.3:   From expert generalist to clinical care director

General practitioner   *Clinical care director*

- Assessment of complaint   Assessment of presenting issue
- Diagnosis   Definition and description
- Investigation   Supporting evidence
- Referral   Seeking specialist advice
- Delegation   Teamworking
- Letter writing   Negotiation of care package
- Pick up the pieces   Co-ordination of care provision
- Recipient of others' problems   Control of resources

Rather than expect the GP to be a font of all wisdom and interpreter, in a limited time, of all the relevant factors in the circumstances of the individual consulting him or her, we can foresee the general practitioner directing the care package that each consultee receives. This may mean referral, delegation or working with therapists to design and implement appropriate packages of care. Directing implies controlling the resources necessary for that package of care and having responsibility for the quality of that care and performance managing the delivery of it. This powerful role would seem to fit best with the forces acting on the general practitioner at this stage.

Registration with the GP – the medical card, the registered list, capitation payments, etc. – has been the currency of power in general practice up until the current time. Unfortunately registration has failed.to balance the rights and responsibilities of the registered patient and the general practitioner. Elements of dependency, carried through from the days before the NHS, have failed to provide an appropriate balance to the relationship. The rising tide of complaints about GPs in the 1990s led to a reform of the complaints process, but evaluation of its successor system[2] has shown us that there is still considerable dissatisfaction with the process from all sides. In addition GPs' power to determine the pattern of health service provision on behalf of their patients has always meant that they are at risk of being criticised by patients, public health, health authorities and hospital trusts for concentrating on some elements of their job, and some of their patients' priorities, and ignoring others. To expect the GP to not only be the jack of all trades, but also the master of them and conductor of the whole orchestra may be asking too much.

Assessing the health needs of the population means more than just interpreting the needs of individual patients, but also more than the formal process of needs analysis, consultation and working with patient interest groups. Balancing the public health responsibilities of GPs with their responsibility for the individual patient consulting them may be improved if consideration is given by PCTs to membership. The extent to which the care available to the community is driven by the *need* (ability to benefit) of the local population, and the extent to which GPs are empowered to determine those needs and the pattern of care, should be considered. If a PCT becomes a membership organisation, i.e. one that is driven by the needs of its members, and whose members are empowered in that relationship, then the role of the GP as being dependent on patient patronage and registration may change. In Choice First the use of personal investment accounts emphasises this trend while in the Feel Good Factor the committee and community spirit have meant that the role of the GP as the holder of the registered list has been consigned to history. It is noteworthy that current government proposals for the establishment of 'foundation hospital trusts' include the adoption of a membership – where staff and local people can choose to become members of the trust, elect its governing board and enjoy the rights and responsibilities of membership. The analogy for PCTs is clear – earn the freedom for local control by the membership.

PCTs are currently struggling with the concepts of partnership with patients, PALS, patient participation groups and working with the voluntary sector. Each of these can be considered as elements of a changing relationship between the PCT, the community and individual citizens which the stakeholders need to be happy with, and which GPs will need to have confidence in, if they are to feel comfortable with moves away from registration.

The role of the GP as gatekeeper to the rest of health and social care, be it through referral, delegation, certification or validating access to a range of services such as social benefit, life insurance, private health insurance benefits, etc., may no longer be wholly appropriate. Gatekeeping has been seen as a very effective way of ensuring the efficiency of healthcare delivery in a resource constrained NHS. GPs have varied greatly in the extent to which they have acted as regulators of access, e.g. to prescription medicines or specialist care, but the gatekeeper function has been seen as one of the prime advantages of the NHS in international comparisons.[3]

As PCTs are developing, the concept of a GP as universal gatekeeper is being challenged by the changing patterns of care, where patients may access NHS Direct, walk-in centres or a range of other primary care providers, such as pharmacists, counsellors, physiotherapists, etc. direct – without being referred through their GPs. The control this gives individual patients over their own personal care and the freedom it offers them to act in their own interests may be empowering, but it also challenges the GP's gatekeeper role. In addition, as the proportion of the national resource that is taken up with funding the health system expands in the early part of the twenty-first century, so the requirement for strict gatekeeping may reduce. Rather we may be looking to GPs to empower and facilitate patients in accessing care which is appropriate to their needs. Constantly blaming GPs for prescribing expensive medicines may be replaced by the requirement for them to meet the requirements of the NSF and disease prevention. In addition, access to social benefits, health insurance and specialist care may have biased the relationship between the GP and his or her individual patients in such a way as to promote 'patronising paternalism'. The need for PCTs to tackle 'the inverse care law'[4] and focus on those in the community in greatest need of healthcare rather than on those who demand it, means that they will need to review the fairness of the gatekeeping system. Encouraging GPs to turn away from the kind, affluent, worried well in favour of the disruptive, socially excluded and needy members of the community will require more leverage and incentives, or a more physiological and systems approach, than 'gatekeeper' symbolises.

The independence of GPs, i.e. as self-employed, self-regulating, employer and capitaliser of their own small business, may need to be curtailed and amended by PCTs if they are to emphasise the important role of GPs as members of the care providing team, with important roles in directing care and enabling patients to access treatment for their health needs. Rather than being isolated and independent from the rest of the health service, GPs need to become central determinants of the health service, and directors of individual care packages (*see* above). In doing so PCTs will need to encourage them to move from an isolationist and independent stance, to a stance which encourages and focuses on their interdependence with other members of the primary care team, and the rest of the healthcare system.

In the new dynamic of the PCT world, leverage for the change in role that the above implies will need to be developed by PCTs. There must be a move away from GPs' income and focus being derived from capitation payments, gatekeeping and expert generalism and towards a situation where their income is dependent on the extent to which they meet the health needs of their population, tackle the inverse care law within their community, enabling the local membership of the organisation to live healthier lives, and effectively directing the care provision provided by them and their team. The challenge for PCTs will be to develop relationships with their GP in such a way as to develop this new dynamic and the income leverage to deliver it.

In essence these arguments mean integrating the role of the GP into the 'managed primary care system'[5] that is evolving in the United Kingdom. The key relationships between GPs and the rest of the stakeholders in that managed care system are changing to support its development and PCTs (in England) and their equivalent in other countries are major stakeholders in this process. The performance management framework of the NHS, whereby national priorities are addressed through the Department of Health, SHAs, NHS trusts, etc., is a powerful framework for changing practice and ensuring that GPs are brought within the managed care framework outlined above.

As discussed in Chapters 5 and 6 an appreciation of the *physiology* as well as the *anatomy* can be helpful if we are to understand how integration of GPs into the managed care system will work and improve the quality of care that patients receive. Simply introducing contracting for primary care, performance appraisal and review, career planning, etc. will not work any more than deciding that waiting lists will be abolished. Rather, PCTs will need to balance their approach by demonstrating that they understand the GP's role 'as a whole' and appreciate the dynamics of the 'system' that he or she works within and often conducts. In each of the archetypes described in Chapter 5 the effect of any change is to induce a counterbalancing result. In seeking to end the 'isolated independent' stance of GPs and encourage the evolution of each of the elements of their professional roles described above, PCTs will need to work with local GPs on all elements of the evolution of their role. This work will need to be undertaken within the context of all the elements of professionalism discussed above, e.g. self-regulation, professional registration, and has to ensure that any changes to the roles and conduct of practitioners are consistent with their professional 'code of conduct'. For GPs these are determined by the General Medical Council.[6] This marks the counterbalance to the flexibility of the local managed care systems, by introducing a strict national framework saying what is expected of GPs, produced by the body which regulates and quality assures the overall standards within the medical profession.

The same kind of forces which are introducing new roles to GPs are also operating on all the other professions involved in providing primary care services. We shall briefly consider how the role of the primary care nurse and primary care pharmacist is developing, but the same could also be said of counsellors, physiotherapists, managers, and dieticians, chiropodists, etc. as they are also exposed to the social and cultural dynamics concerned.

Nursing

Nurses working in the primary care sector have until recently been largely concerned with the personal care of individuals. This care may have been provided within general practice (practice nurse) or in a community clinic or in the patient's home (district nursing). In the past much of the personal care involved chronic disease management, convalescent care, wound care and management of varicose ulcers. It was within a professional paradigm which emphasised support and dependency, professional detachment and patient instruction rather than promoting patient autonomy. It emphasised teamworking across organisational boundaries, e.g. hospital, social services, etc., to a greater extent than for GPs. Nurses who have developed their professional role as health visitors, occupational health nurses and, increasingly, as practice nurses have chosen to develop and emphasise the important role of nurses as promoters of individual health. Rather than a model, or paradigm, emphasising dependency this is a paradigm which emphasises patient autonomy and encourages nurses to see themselves as educators of patients and empowerers of patients, helping them to lead more independent and fulfilling lives.

Over the last two decades of the twentieth century the development of the nursing profession, its separation and independence from the medical profession and the emergence of nursing as a force within the healthcare sector has been a strong theme. One of the levers for these changes has been strong management. Nursing has always had elements of hierarchy within its professional structures, e.g. matron, but the efficient administration, management and delivery of care cannot just rely on performance management through hierarchy. In addition to a hierarchy there is a need for a *currency*, if leverage is to be effectively developed. Over the last 20 years in the nursing profession that currency has been the 'nursing process'. The introduction of formal instruments such as nursing reports, nursing records, care plans, etc. has served to demonstrate, develop and formalise the professional behaviour of nurses. In the new century this process needs to evolve from being a paper-based and formal, if rather rigid, structure to become a system supporting the professional roles and identities of nurses. In doing so, the nursing process has to reflect the role of the nurse as the 'care manager'. As a care manager the nurse has responsibility not only for the personal care of her patients, but also for ensuring that his or her individual needs are met, co-ordinated and delivered in such a way as to encourage the patient's autonomy, personal responsibility and development. The nurse may well be working within protocols and guidelines, e.g. NHS Direct, or working as part of a team and only responsible for part of the overall care package that a patient is receiving. The extent to which nurses are managers of the patient's overall care will vary, but the nursing process has to adapt and become more coherent with those providing the other elements of care. Common records with the GP, team meetings across organisational and professional boundaries to co-ordinate care, the development of instruments to manage the quality of care provided by the team and opening up the nursing and other professions to assessment and quality assurance processes across professional boundaries will all be important.

The culture of nursing over the twentieth century has been largely reactive. Nurses have reacted to referral or delegation from the medical profession, to social or military disaster, e.g. world wars, and to the consequences of disease and famine, e.g. epidemics and refugees. In the twenty-first century it is becoming apparent that nurses need to assert themselves a little more. Rather than simply reacting to the circumstances that they work within they are being encouraged to become more proactive. This includes seeing themselves as enablers and empowerers of individual responsibility as described above, but also as important instruments for implementing community policy. It has been apparent for many years that immunisation, breast feeding, weight reduction, smoking cessation and exercise are all activities that help people live healthier lives. If nurses are to do more than just simply exhort and encourage those they care for to implement each of these health promoting activities then they will need to develop *leverage*[7] through working within the managed care system outlined above.

Pharmacists

Earlier parts of this book looked at the history of the community pharmacist in the primary care sector and described the forces that have led to their current professional role as dispenser, therapeutics adviser, small shopkeeper and external safety net for prescribing. As a result of the social, technological, economic and cultural forces operating on the profession at the beginning of the twenty-first century these roles are evolving and changing.

- The requirement for the pharmacist to be the dispenser of medicines and to act in a professional manner in doing so is reducing. The introduction of strict quality assurance of medicines through instruments such as the Medicines Control Agency (MCA) and the introduction of original pack dispensing through blister packs, has reduced the risks of the dispensing process and the need for the pharmacist to manufacture pills, make up medicines and lotions, and dispense bespoke products according to the patient's individual prescription. The emergence of the modern therapeutic armoury and the strong pharmaceutical industry has meant that the dispensing role is having to change. Rather, the dispenser needs to become a *medicines manager*. The medicines manager will use the professional skills and training of his or her pharmacy background to become the patient's medicine manager. This role will involve the pharmacist in ensuring the patient's access to the medicine he or she needs, e.g. through electronic prescribing and the development of delivery systems, ensuring compliance with treatment regimes through aids and devices, monitoring effectiveness of medication, e.g. reducing the risk for patients from their medicines. With the development of *pharmacogenetics* the pharmacist will increasingly become a guardian or protector of patients, ensuring that the medicines that they receive are appropriate for their genetic heritage.
- Traditionally pharmacists have been consulted by individual customers about their health problems and have screened or advised patients whether to go to casualty, their GP or self-medicate. As their role evolves they have become, in the hospital setting, much more concerned with supporting the rest of the care providing team in ensuring that the therapeutic armoury at their disposal is used effectively. Integrating the community pharmacist into the primary care team may well encourage more effective use of medicines by that team and the provision of higher quality care to individual patients. As the dispensing role of pharmacists declines, so the need for community pharmacists to become part of the primary care team and offer their expertise in therapeutics and clinical pharmacy practice to the team is increasing. The extent to which the clinical pharmacist can take responsibility for issues such as anticoagulation control, diabetic monitoring and other aspects of the monitoring of drug therapy is currently uncertain. Certainly pharmacists have many of the skills and the understanding of treatments which will

be necessary for effective monitoring of treatments and if they work within the primary care team in areas where their expertise is appropriate, acknowledged and developed then this clinical pharmacy role could be very valuable.

- Personal ownership of the pharmacy premises by community pharmacists has been in decline for many years. Corporatisation of community pharmacy through supermarket chains and multiples has meant a decline in the fortunes of the small shopkeeper/independent pharmacist. Increasingly, community pharmacists are salaried employees who work within the management frameworks of their company and whose independent advice to customers has to reflect the ethics and values of the company they work for. The challenge to the PCTs and the primary care team will be to develop the expertise of the community pharmacist as an agent for managing the care that patients receive through the trust and team and to work with them and their employers to agree how their expertise will be developed and adapted to meet the needs of the community.

- The prescribing system within the United Kingdom where the doctor signs the prescription and the pharmacist acts as a check to ensure that the prescription is safe and appropriate has been important as the therapeutics revolution of the last 50 years has developed. Computerised prescribing, electronic dispensing and increasing availability of medicines without prescription has meant that this system with the pharmacist as 'external safety net' is in need of review. Rather the role needs to evolve to become an adviser to the prescriber and the rest of the primary care team about all aspects of medicines management and therapeutics so that the increasingly sophisticated and complex care packages that patients need can be safely delivered and monitored.

The above considerations, which could be extended to other care providing professions, illustrate how the forces acting on professional behaviour have been leading, are leading and can be anticipated to lead to new definitions and descriptions of professional behaviour.

Implications of the future

In appreciating the dynamics of Choice First and the Feel Good Factor we have to reflect that each marks a considerable challenge for the concepts of professionalism within the primary care sector. The implications discussed above for general practitioners, nurses and pharmacists are profound and many existing practitioners find them difficult to accept. In both of the futures the current changes in professional attitudes and behaviour have evolved further.

- For general practitioners there is the transition to becoming directors and primary care physicians in Choice First. This role will involve the management of complex pathology, the direction of the business and the co-ordination of care packages involving a range of clinicians. While gatekeeping, registration, expert generalism and independence have been left behind, the value of the professional adviser to members and as a specialist in the management of complex pathology has developed. With so much care being provided through Choice First and so little being referred to secondary care, the responsibilities of the primary care physician are greater than for current GPs. He or she will work closely with specialists working outside hospital and may well have important responsibilities in areas of special expertise. In the Feel Good Factor the role of the GP is similarly unrecognisable compared to the current day. With radical change to professional education at both pre-registration and continuing professional development levels there is integration of roles and career progression for individuals who work in the primary care team. While general medical practice continues to look after the majority of pathology in the community, the major role has become the prevention of disease and the support of health promoting activity in the community. New technology has enabled much of care to be transferred from the hospital to the home base setting and local teams have responsibility for providing this care. The performance management of teams rather than individuals means a very different professional paradigm for GPs.

- Nursing within the two futures shows a similar divide. In Choice First nurses and the nursing process have become involved with the provision of acute care, the promotion of healthy living and the implementation of evidence based medicine. Chronic disease management of the weak and vulnerable is less of a priority for the organisation and the traditional caring role of nursing has been consigned to history. In the Feel Good Factor nursing can be expected to play a pivotal role in the locality teams and, because of the universal provision ethic of this future, we can anticipate that personal care of the elderly, vulnerable and weak will be more of a priority.

- Community pharmacy has developed in the Choice First future to be a vital part of the evidence-based practice provided by First Call. Further development of medicine's management and clinical pharmacy in the community has meant that new technologies, as they develop, have expanded the horizons of the primary care sector, but this has only been safe as the therapeutic expertise of pharmacy has been integrated into the rest of care provision. In the Feel Good Factor we can anticipate that some of the team will have specialised in medicine management and that supporting individual patients in making choices about their health and health problems will be an important element.

Reconfiguration of care

During the latter part of the twentieth century much of the traditional role of district general hospitals was transferred into the community. Elderly care has largely been transferred into nursing and residential care homes, sheltered housing and supporting the elderly in their own homes. This has not been without its problems and bed blocking, closure of small nursing and residential care homes and isolation of the elderly in their own homes when their families live far away are all current issues causing concern. Much of mental health provision, including that of the elderly mental infirm, has similarly been transferred from institutionalised care into community care and the emergence of new treatments such as long-acting antipsychotics has changed the mental health paradigm dramatically. Long-stay care of those with learning disabilities has similarly been largely transferred from NHS institutional provision into the community. The average length of stay of individuals with acute illness has also decreased in hospital and increasing proportions of surgery and general medicine are provided as day cases. Each of these transfers of care from hospital into the community has enabled the hospital sector to concentrate on the provision of high-tech specialist care and transferred everything else into the community where it is provided by primary care teams with the support of outreach from the specialsist services. The major reconfiguration of the pattern of care that has been involved has not been complemented by major reconfiguration in the capacity of the primary care and community care sectors to provide that care, or by the transfer of expertise and resources from hospitals to ensure the quality of that care. As a result the volume and complexity of care provided in the home has been a cause of concern to primary care and practitioners and will be a test for PCTs.

As the *community revolution* of the twenty-first century evolves and follows on from the industrial revolution of the nineteenth century and the social revolution of the twentieth century, then a reconfiguration of care can be seen as one of the emerging strands of the revolution. The reconfiguration takes care out of the institutional setting and into specialist and generalist spheres within a community care setting. Specialist practitioners will need to provide that care outside of their traditional institutions, and other professionals within the setting will need to adapt their professionalism and skills to support the range of care that is required. This will change the pattern of healthcare delivery and challenge traditional concepts of health and disease. The development of genetic medicine should enfranchise future generations to make more informed choices about their own and their children's future, but also challenge the interface between individual responsibility and community responsibility. In the two futures, Choice First clarifies the position where individual responsibility is paramount while in the Feel Good Factor it is the community's interest which is paramount. Genetic medicine crystallises the difference between these two futures because in Choice First it is the strong who thrive while in the Feel Good Factor it is the weak who are protected.

Skill substitution

An emerging theme at the beginning of the twenty-first century has been the lack of capacity within the health sector and the requirement to use scarce resources efficiently and effectively. One of the ways that has been developing to conserve scarce professional resources has been to use clinicians with less training to undertake some of the roles traditionally being provided by highly trained practitioners. The emergence of venisectionists, nursing assistants and auxiliary nurses, nursery nurses and pharmacy technicians are all examples. Rather than feel that the GP or district nurse should provide all the personal care that a patient requires, a whole team is now involved with consequential implications for communication and teamworking. We can anticipate that skill substitution will become even more defined as PCTs seek to develop their provider roles within the constraints of a limited number of skilled practitioners. The increasing complexity of care provided within the PCT and the increasing dependency of an elderly and socially isolationist society (with dispersed family structures) will mean primary care teams providing more and more support as time moves on.

Emerging technologies

The history of the primary care sector as outlined earlier in the book has been of development in response to the changing world in which primary care is delivered. Throughout the industrial revolution change was driven by the need for a healthy workforce and the development of medical technology such as anaesthetics. During the social revolution of the twentieth century the sector has evolved in response to the therapeutics revolution and the major changes in demography, education and the breakdown of rigid social structures. The development of new transport and communication technologies has also had a major effect on the primary care sector by ensuring that the whole population has access to information about health and that social mobility has challenged long-term caring relationships as well as increasing the requirement for care providers to be available and responsive to patient demand at all times.

As the sector moves into the twenty-first century these evolutionary forces will not go away and we can anticipate further developments in each of the above areas. A few of these areas will be considered in a little more detail, with reference made to the two primary care futures and how they illustrate the themes.

Supervision

The emergence of video surveillance – of traffic congestion, shopping centre crowds, airports and cash machines – has been driven by issues of public safety and public security. In the primary care sector the safety of isolated vulnerable elderly has been promoted by the use of personal alarm buzzers linked to the telephone system in the same way as baby alarms work for worried parents. The possibility that such surveillance may make it safe for the process of the de-institutionalisation (*see* above) to evolve further so as to permit the elderly to stay longer in their own homes, the sick to be cared for away from the institutional risks from cross-infection and parents to feel safer in caring for their children and babies has to be considered very likely as it meets the criterion of increasing safety and security, as well as being an efficient use of resources.

As well as video surveillance the possibility of the monitoring of biological functions at a distance is likely to develop further. We already have tagging of prisoners when on weekend release or to avoid sending offenders to jail and we also have 24-hour monitoring of blood pressure and cardiac rhythm. The possibility of radio or telephonic monitoring of other physiological functions 'at a distance' is being considered. Many of the rather artificial functions of hospitals such as EEG, lung function and biochemical monitoring of blood glucose in diabetics or anticoagulant monitoring are under consideration.

In Choice First we can see how First Call's array of videophones can facilitate diagnosis and treatment 'at a distance' and how attractive would be the efficiencies of telemetry-based diagnostics and monitoring to the board. Such monitoring would reduce dependence on institutional specialist secondary care and, along with the emerging new treatments to replace surgical intervention, has made it possible for 'bed days' to be reduced to less than 10% of current practice.

In the Feel Good Factor tele-links to the 'phys rehab centre' enable local staff to manage most patient problems. The ethos is supporting individual citizens in making choices, taking control of their own lives and acting responsibly. The use of video surveillance, telemetry, etc. will be supported by the committee even if it is a little intrusive because it helps to promote individual citizens' autonomy and helps them live healthier lives.

Workforce development

The emerging responsibilities of the primary care workforce are described above and further illustrated by Choice First and the Feel Good Factor. PCTs will need to work with their workforce so that they can adapt to the new responsibilities as they emerge and develop. Developing the current workforce as well as training those entering the workforce will be made much easier if full use is made of modern technology to support individuals and teams with their development. The full range of multimedia approaches will be required and will include:

- paper-based material as many in the current workforce will be most comfortable with this format
- audio and video tape material

- use of lectures, workshops and other dynamic and interactive formats, particularly for discussion and challenge
- the Internet. The provision of learning material via the Internet and the use of the Internet to support discussion, feedback and interaction can be expected to develop further. New technology also permits much greater access to information and support of the workforce and citizens in using that information to best advantage. An early example is the use of computerised decision support by NHS Direct in order to provide a triage service and increasingly to provide a single point of entry and advice for patients accessing the primary care sector.

The emerging theme is of technology supporting the development of learning by individuals, teams and organisations. Chapter 4 looked at some of the dimensions that primary care would need to address in becoming a learning system and it is likely that the innovative use of technological support will promote PCTs in addressing these responsibilities.

In the Feel Good Factor close monitoring of practice by computer-based systems is used as a performance management tool and as a quality development tool by the Bureau. As practitioners work through their training programmes and as they support citizens in taking more control over their own lives so the use of technological support becomes more vital. At its core this organisation is a community development organisation and will harness all supportive technologies towards that purpose. In developing its workforce the Bureau can be expected to lean heavily on technology for both provision and quality assurance.

In Choice First technology drives service provision and can be expected also to underpin workforce development. With such a strong quality of care ethic in the organisation it can be anticipated that First Call will invest heavily in maintaining up-to-date education and training programmes for all grades of staff and see it as an essential prerequisite for attracting and maintaining its market share and membership.

Accessing information

Throughout the development of healthcare during the twentieth century the existence of a lifelong record, maintained in primary care by the individual's practitioner, has been one of the key features of the UK's managed care system. The maintenance of individual confidentiality has often meant the development of separate health records by each practitioner caring for a patient with all the inefficiencies of duplication and risk of each record being inadequate. It remains important, however, that personal confidential information is respected and not available for use without the consent of the individual citizens. It is widely accepted that technology will enable a unified individual record to be maintained across all sectors of healthcare and this has been explored through the electronic patient record projects which have been running for several years in hospital and in primary care. General practice has moved a long way away from the traditional paper-based 'Lloyd George' record towards computerised systems and has encouraged, employed and attached primary care team staff to join in using this common record. Links with the hospital sector have been more disjointed, but technology should enable direct transfer of information between the sectors – it is already doing so for e-mail and pathology reports, and this can be expected to grow. The issue of the security and confidentiality of this information is important and new technological approaches are needed if the systems are to be trustworthy. The holding of very confidential information, such as an individual's HIV and genetic status, or his or her emotional, physical and spiritual histories make it vital that people can trust the security of the record and that they control access to it.

In Choice First access to the record is controlled via the use of pin numbers and iris technology. We can see that this is already being used as a passport control aid at major airports and might anticipate it spreading to regulating access to health records. The control via pin numbers, when the individual is not physically present for iris scanning, is already widely used for regulating access to bank accounts and can be expected to be adapted for accessing medical records.

In the Feel Good Factor, while the issue of technological regulation of records is not directly dealt with, we can expect that the balance between the community's interest as opposed to the individual's interest will be more tipped towards the former. The Bureau is likely to see that the rights of the individual to confidentiality at all times will come second to the community's interest and that of the greater good of the public. The Bureau may wish to pressurise individuals to have immunisations, to stop smoking or otherwise abusing their bodies and to take part in community development activities. To this extent the individual's right to maintain absolute control over access to his or her records will be more limited.

Pathology tests

Pathology has been at the forefront of technological development over the last 20 years and we can expect that the trend will continue. Technology can support the development of new tests, new ways of performing tests and new ways of communication about the results and implication of tests. Tests that can be undertaken without invasive procedures, such as blood sampling or buccal swabs for DNA sampling, have developed, as well as entirely new tests to increase the certainty of diagnosis, and genetic testing in histopathology. It is increasingly frustrating for primary care practitioners and patients to have to wait days and sometimes weeks for the results of tests which take only a few minutes to perform. Delays in the cervical cytology screening programme are a particular cause for concern, but the issue also applies to other results with implications for the future health of the patient concerned. There are two alternative approaches to improving the efficiency of the system by the introduction of new technology.

1 Communications within the system are improved so that district based laboratories in secondary care can deliver results within a time frame which is acceptable to patients and primary care practitioners.
2 The development of *near patient testing* is boosted in the United Kingdom. This technology has developed more rapidly in Europe and the rest of the developed world and would enable a considerable proportion of pathology testing to be undertaken in the primary care sector. Monitoring of glucose by diabetic patients has developed in the UK, but self-monitoring of anticoagulation and other areas of monitoring and diagnostics are less developed.

With so much care provided in the primary care sector in Choice First and the Feel Good Factor, we can anticipate that much of the district general hospital's pathology service will have been transferred into First Call and the Bureau. While this will have been driven by the demands of membership in Choice First, it will have been more centrally driven by the performance management framework and modernisation trends in the Feel Good Factor.

Evolution

While much of this chapter has been seeking to explore current issues from the perspective of the heritage and the two futures, it should be appreciated that we are dealing with dynamic processes. The evolution of the professional paradigms has been over succeeding generations and change to those paradigms, driven largely by social factors and technological change, will be gradual. The reconfiguration of care can only be successfully implemented through a process of rc-engineering and consensual project working through programmes like NHS collaboratives, PMS piloting and guideline developments. These are all time-consuming processes and the pace will be relatively slow as the pressure of day-to-day care provision and the challenge of change both get in the way of practitioner commitments. Similarly the change to being a health sector driven by the needs of its membership rather than by the convenience of its providers will not happen rapidly. For generations the heritage of gatekeeping, patronising paternalism and registration has affected relationships, values and attitudes between primary care and the population. Developing a sector which is centred around the needs of patients and is driven by the views and needs of all citizens, i.e. its membership, will be evolutionary and follow on as a response to the forces discussed not only in this chapter but in the rest of the book. Technological change is also evolutionary. While the pace of technological change may have quickened over the last century individuals will always take some time to adapt their approach and test out technological change before becoming committed to it. The phrase 'technology changes ground rules' is however important. The implication is that technological change can change the way we think about fundamental issues, challenge our underpinning values, change the relationship between stakeholders and change the paradigms of care much more rapidly than political, economic or demographic forces.

It is worth reiterating that the effect of these issues and of the discussions in earlier chapters is to redefine the purpose of the primary care sector and wider health service. Rather than being a disease management service which has evolved over the last half of the twentieth century to efficiently manage acute and chronic disease, the NHS is becoming much more of a health service. The focus is on maintaining and improving health, avoiding disease and promoting healthy lifestyles. The pre-eminence of the medical model, based as it is on disease centred paradigms, is being challenged. Rather the service is focusing on community and personal development, promoting individual autonomy and asking questions about the relevance of its heritage. The danger is that in rightly doing so, the balance will be tipped too far in the direction of personal and community development and the lessons of the past will be forgotten:

- the importance of *trust, care* and *support*
- the importance of disease management when individuals are sick, infirm, frail or dependent
- the importance of advice and personal care at times of distress
- the heritage of expert generalism where family doctors can make balanced judgements across all the factors relevant to an individual's consultation rather than being focused on the presenting problem or the personal development of the individual.

What is required is a more balanced approach to the themes emerging at the present time and in appreciation of how the heritage of the past can inform the development of the primary care sector for the future. The agreement to increased investment in the NHS, allied to programmes of change management and modernisation, sends important signals to the primary care sector. The national plan[8] and its implementation programmes, national agencies and local boards have been helping to set the strategic framework and approach to many of the themes outlined in this chapter. The use of tools, such as NHS collaboratives, learning networks, leadership programmes, personal learning accounts, cancer and genetics networks, new training schemes for doctors, nurses, etc. is an asset. In addition there will be a need for planning, development and management to be based much more than at present on the teams – often from different institutions – who care for patients and users in their journey through the system. This means a much greater focus on systems than on individual consultations and on care provided by teams over time rather than reacting to individual problems as they present. The challenge for PCTs will be to implement this modernisation agenda within their own organisations and across the boundaries with other stakeholders without losing the confidence of the workforce or the local population.

References

1 Gillam S and Meads G (2001) *Modernisation and the Future of General Practice.* King's Fund, London.
2 Posnet J *et al.* (2001) *NHS Complaints Procedure, National Evaluation.* York Health Economics Consortium and System Three Social Research.
3 Starfield B (1994) Is primary care essential? *Lancet.* **344**: 1129–33.
4 Tudor Hart J (1998) *A New Kind of Doctor.* Merlin Press, London.
5 Meads G and Ashcroft J (2000) *Relationships in the NHS – bridging the gap.* Royal Society of Medicine, London.
6 General Medical Council (1998) *Maintaining Good Medical Practice.* GMC, London.
7 Senge PM (1993) *The Fifth Discipline.* Random House Business Books, New York.
8 Department of Health (2000) *The NHS Plan Implementation Programme.* DoH, London.

CHAPTER 10

Summary and conclusions

This chapter will not seek to summarise all the themes and issues which have been explored in previous chapters. They stand on their own as the constituents of this book and the determinants of the conclusions that this chapter will suggest. The chapter will consider the following suggestions, which are also summarised in Tables 10.1–10.5.

- Implications for the system both internal to primary care and external to it.
- The extent to which primary care can be regarded as 'fit for the future'.
- The future of primary care as a system.
- The implications of the modernisation agenda for primary care and the rest of the NHS.

We have to reflect that health is a dynamic process and the system for providing healthcare is similarly a dynamic process or *system*. Individual health and the health providing system are each made up of episodes or events, to an extent predetermined by heritage or inheritence and to an extent at the mercy of external events. In both individual health and the health providing system it is the relationship between issues and events rather than the issues or events themselves that are the major determinants of what happens. The biographical or lifetime focus of the primary care sector can provide a wealth of examples to illustrate this.

Box 10.1:   Case study – Meg and Jim

Meg and Jim celebrated their golden wedding last year. They are both in their late seventies and in pretty good health. Meg has always been a worrier and her aches and pains, anxieties and mild hypertension concern her. She also worries about Jim who has severe arthritis in his knees, is a bit forgetful and has always drunk more than she would want.

   Meg and Jim represent the centre of a large family with over 40 children, grandchildren and great grandchildren, cousins, nieces, nephews, etc. Each member of the extended family owes a proportion of their identity to Meg and Jim and in their various ways acknowledges the debt that they owe them. Their own health biographies reveal their daughter's obesity and hypertension with mild diabetes and consequent eye and kidney complications. Son-in-law Brian's addiction to cigarettes and the stress of modern life have led to early retirement on health grounds as well as chairmanship of the allotment society and a tendency to playing the wrong notes on the organ in church. Sadly granddaughter Diana died from cystic fibrosis, but her brothers and sisters, Christopher, Daisy, Thomas and James, are growing up fast to maintain the family traditions of exuberance, intelligence and individualism. One or more may be carriers of cystic fibrosis, but they otherwise seem pretty normal. The other members of the extended family have had a full range of health problems from difficulties in conceiving to senile dementia, from HIV to cancer and from depression to autism.

The relationships between the family members and between them and the community that they live in, including its healthcare providers, law enforcers and teachers are what determine the future of the family and Meg and Jim's contentment as they look forward to their diamond anniversary.

Internal implications

Table 10.1 looks at the implications of the issues considered in this book to the internal members of the primary care system. We shall consider each line separately.

Table 10.1:   Implications for the system – internal

Who for	From	To
Patients	Supplicants	Members
Carers	Exploitation	Control
Pharmacists	Pill pushers	Therapy managers
Nurses	Personal care	Primary provider
GPs	Jack of all trades	Primary care physician
		Care co-ordinator
General manager	Control	Support
PAMs	Delegation	Team worker
	Peripheralisation	
Practice manager	Employee	Quality assurance
	GP's agent	Communicator
Practice	Islands	Archipelagos

Patients

The previous relationship between individual patients and the primary care system has been primarily one of supplication. Patients have been the passive recipients of *patronising paternalism*, the recipients of nursing care and obliged to the community pharmacist for his dispensing of their prescriptions. In the future they will become participating and active *members* in the development of their own health and contentment. They will individually determine how and through what processes that health is determined and control to a much greater extent the policies and plans of the professionals making up the primary care systems and the organisations directing and controlling the sector. Membership implies much more than a holding of an NHS membership card, but a full range of rights and responsibilities detailing the relationship between the citizen and the primary care healthcare system.[1]

Carers

For many years those who provide personal care to the sick have had to find fulfilment in the gratitude of their patients. Family members will often face economic difficulties in giving up work to care. Voluntary support for caring has depended on altruism and nursing on the commitment and vocation of its professional practitioners. The healthcare system has exploited these carers and taken for granted their commitment to an extent that is no longer sustainable. In the modern world economic, demographic and social constraints mean that family and voluntary caring is often tainted by resentment and the vocation of nursing has evolved into a modern professionalism more focused on assessment, care management and advocacy. The implications for the future must be that the system has to value personal carers in a way which permits and encourages the kind of care which the community needs. Most carers are not interested in being rewarded monetarily so long as they are not penalised for caring – but they frequently say that they would like:

- more control over the care package that is being provided
- more control over the extent of their own commitment and
- more control over the policies and procedures of the primary and specialist care team which is supporting them.

If the primary care system is to retain and foster the rich heritage of commitment and voluntary sector activity that has characterised the development of welfare services in the UK, then it must realise that the changing culture of society requires change to these relationships.

Pharmacists

The separation of the profession of pharmacy from medicine before and during the industrial revolution was based on the manufacturing, dispensing and science of therapeutics. The small business ethic and the street corner access and support service was vital for the economic success of community pharmacy, and the battles for territory with dispensing pharmacies and supermarkets have moulded and predetermined some current attitudes. With the rise of the global pharmaceutical industry, original pack dispensing, electronic prescribing and Internet based supply of medicines, the practice of community pharmacy is facing hard choices and in truth the current arrangements are probably economically and socially unsustainable. There is, however, a great need for primary care organ-isations, and the patients they represent, to have a much greater understanding of medicines management and therapeutics than in the past.

Community pharmacists will move their professionalism into being therapy managers: advisers to the medical and nursing professions on therapeutics and to patients on how to manage their medicines. Allied to this medicines manage-ment role there are several other areas where their expertise could be further developed towards:

- monitoring treatment which has to vary over time, such as anticoagulation
- screening for markers of disease, such as diabetes and hypertension
- advising on the appropriateness of medication, for example in the field of pharmacogenetics
- advising on the benefits and risks involved in using recreational drugs, what-ever their legislative status.

Nurses

The implications for all the branches of the nursing profession is a move from being:

- the personal carer; the professional most closely involved with the care of the long-term chronic sick
- the person who looks after them through the trauma of childbirth and into parenthood and who supports them through convalescence.

And a move to a role which respects their autonomy and professionalism, but asks questions of their heritage of vocation and service.

Specialist nursing roles and practice in areas such as dialysis, neurology, asthma, diabetes, etc. have developed to support skill substitution within the medical model. The development of processes such as nurse triage, nurse prescribing, walk-in centres and NHS Direct are attempts to refocus the professionalism of nursing in primary care towards being the patient's agent in health as well as in disease. The trend is to develop the primary care nurse as the patient's main primary care provider and increasingly their first point of call when they are seeking health advice or treatment. This is an example of skill substitution with the nurse as the first point of contact and referral through the nurse to the other professions in primary care, such as doctors, pharmacists, counsellors, etc.

General practitioners

As discussed in the two primary care futures and throughout this book, the role of the GP as the 'jack of all trades' has been changing rapidly through the first 50 years of the health service from the 'Dr Finlay' model of patronising paternal-ism. The redefined role now has to reflect the inappropriateness of some of the fundamental features of its heritage. Registration, gatekeeping, expert generalism and professional partnership no longer seem as well designed for modern circum-stances as they were for the NHS in the post-war years. The future role of the medical practitioner in primary care would seem likely to be based on their role as physicians – diagnoser, pathology manager, care co-ordinator and personal adviser on all matters relating to the management and prevention of disease. In this role there will be a requirement to move with patients through their journey between home and specialist care in order to co-ordinate complex care packages. With the increasing sub-specialisation in institutional based healthcare, such as in hospital, there is an increasing requirement for care co-ordination. In the UK the extent of the separation between hospital practice and general practice has historically been greater than in many other countries. In the USA family physicians will often be involved in hospital based care and the time has probably come to begin dismantling some of the artificial barriers preventing similar approaches to co-ordination of care in the UK. Until now it has been hospital specialists who have sometimes made *domiciliary* visits, perhaps the time has come for primary care physicians to do *hospital* visits.

General managers

The introduction of general management into the health service during the 1970s[2] has done much to encourage the evolution and development of the primary care sector, and to foster a system which is designed to be safe for the community to trust its resources to, and have confidence in. The core skills of general management do, however, now need to reflect on the changing world illustrated in Choice First and the Feel Good Factor. The specialist areas of human resource management, financial management, planning and estates manage-ment continue to be important, but the extent to which they control and direct the whole system should now be questioned. If general management has been efficient not just at administration of the primary care system, but also at the interface between central control and political imperatives around waiting times, financial balance and quality assurance, then the risk is leaving competent general managers vulnerable and exposed when faced with the cold winds of political change, efficiency savings or competing clinical priorities. What is required is clinically credible and knowledgeable direction and management of the system. The primary care sector, as it becomes more corporate in its approach, has to reflect on its heritage and values and ensure that its decision-making processes are driven by clinical management imperatives to a greater extent than general management imperatives.

PAMs

Physiotherapists, occupational therapists, chiropodists, etc. have all played a supportive role to the medical model in the first 50 years of the NHS. Often employed by community trusts or working as private sector contractors, they have been largely peripheral to the medical approach to healthcare. As the provision of care has moved out of hospital into the community and as more and more complex packages are provided in the home, so the need for integration between all the members of the primary care team (including PAMs) must mean that PAMs become more integrated into the primary care team. Their approach of maintaining the individual's independence and autonomy alongside the practical skills that they bring fits in well with the emerging roles of primary care physicians and nurses. Many are now employed by PCTs and within both the futures – Choice First and the Feel Good Factor – we can see how breaking down the barriers between the professional paradigms could contribute to a much more effective future provision of healthcare.

Practice managers

The leadership of small primary care teams, their co-ordination and the management of the business have led to the emergence of a whole range of approaches to being a 'practice manager'. Highly skilled and multitalented though many of them are, their focus has always been on the practice. Being employees of the business and therefore of the GPs who own and run the business they have never had the power within the organisation to direct it. Rather their role has been to implement the policies of the GPs and effectively to administer the organisation. As the role of the practice changes, towards being part of the PCT and away from being the building blocks forming the architecture of primary care, so the role of the practice manager has to become less focused internally on the business of the practice and more focused externally on ensuring that the organisation meets the needs of the local community and responds to the direction of the PCT.

Practices

The traditional model of the separate 'island' practice no longer reflects the nature of healthcare delivery in the twenty-first century. While the practice model has much to commend it in terms of sensitivity, flexibility, accessibility and responsiveness, it is not a model that has sufficient elements of quality assurance, corporate governance, efficiency and effectiveness to survive in its current form. Practices increasingly need to work with other practices if they are to plan and co-ordinate care across the whole community, be trusted with the control of the majority of health service resources and have the skills necessary to provide the complex care packages which patients require. Islands need to become archipelagos so that each individual island is linked to its surrounding ones if the whole population is to be effectively cared for. The requirement is for all the professionals and staff to see themselves as part of the archipelago and consider how they can develop themselves and their services through this broader range of relationships.

The traditional 'partnership', with GP principals as partners, owners of the premises, employers of the staff, main care providers and directors, has to evolve to reflect the changing responsibilities of the practice – its multiprofessional primary care team needs to be more involved in decision making, it needs to become more open and more responsive, to be less introverted and less parochial.

This then is the radical set of implications for the constituents of the current primary care system and a summary of some of the ways in which the forces described in this book are moulding current primary care practice.

External implications

Table 10.2 illustrates how the relationship between the primary care sector and its external partners is evolving. As PCTs seek to exert more influence over the whole pattern of healthcare delivery in hospital and at home through their commissioning of care and control of resources, so the dominant role of the hospital and the specialist in the healthcare system is being challenged. Rather, the specialist practitioner and the hospital as an institution are being seen as the servant of the care co-ordinator, the primary care physician and the PCT. The role of specialist care is changing from directing the whole package of care to advising on its specialist aspects and ensuring that the complex needs of patients are individually addressed.

The relationship between the primary care sector and the voluntary sector is also changing. The adaptability and the responsiveness of the voluntary sector has always been a major asset in the NHS and has helped it to be a true provider

Table 10.2: Implications for the system – external

Who for	From	To
Secondary care	Master	Servant
Specialist care	Director	Adviser
Voluntary sector	Gap filler	Partner
Social care	Dartboard	Co-provider
Local authority	Parallel	Co-ordinate
Emergency services	Incidental	Integrated
Health authority	Victim	Co-ordinate
DoH	Doer	Supporter
Finance	SAFF	SVP
	Revenue (+capital)	Revenue/capital
Planning	Annual	Medium term
Politicians	Accountable	Arms length
Drug industry	Cash cow/black hole	Agent

of welfare services rather than just an arm of the welfare state. Unfortunately the voluntary sector has often had to fill the gaps for which state provision has been unable to find the resources, and this has sometimes been a vital instrument of constructive change. The voluntary hospitals reflect this heritage alongside the role of the Red Cross in providing nursing and equipment, the WRVS in providing meals on wheels and the army of voluntary drivers, patient advocates and hospital visitors. Increasingly the corporate development of PCTs requires a strong non-executive element if it is to reflect the needs of the local community. Partnership with the voluntary sector so that the professional providers and the voluntary sector trust each other, and develop their care plans and approach together would seem to provide a more constructive approach for the future.

Increasingly, welfare provision is having to reflect both the health needs of individuals and their social care needs. Separation of social care from healthcare has always been rather artificial, but too many individuals and groups have suffered from the separation in the past. The health needs of those in residential children's homes and the social care needs of the isolated, vulnerable or frail individuals in the community, have thus far been considered separately by social service departments and the health service. The need now is for much greater integration, joint planning, joint financing and joint provision of care and to move the relationship between health and social care from being the *dart and the dartboard* which each throws at the other to discharge their frustrations, to partnership working where each seeks to become a co-provider of welfare services.

If the relationship with social service departments is evolving so also is the relationship with local authorities. In the past health authorities and local authorities often worked in parallel while waving to each other across the street when they passed. There has been little or no effective partnership between the environmental health department of a local authority and the public health department of the health authority; little co-ordination between the planning department's aspirations for community development and the health authority's need to plan healthcare delivery; little co-ordination of the socially excluded and deprived population's services between the police, health services, social services and transport. While the future in Choice First sees health as a specialist independent community service, in the Feel Good Factor the Bureau is operating more as an arm of local democracy.

It would seem that, with the establishment of SHAs, the NHS still sees its future as separate from other more democratic community organisations – such as local authorities and regional assemblies. Continuing to direct PCTs through a framework of national imperatives and accountability agreements looks doomed to failure. Rather, moves towards being more responsive to local communities, more accountable to them and more open to influence by them should be encouraged. SHAs should become departments of regional government with PCTs absorbing environmental health and social services to become autonomous welfare agencies reporting to local authority welfare committees.

Similarly there are implications for other external relationships between the primary care sector and its partners in providing emergency services and in becoming part of an integrated system where all the roles and responsibilities are changing. It may well be that the increasing power of the PCT will push longer term planning out of the rigidity of the SAFF mechanisms, out of the rigid separation of revenue and capital funding and out of the model which sees the provision of healthcare as a political football and towards a model which sees health as an individual, personal responsibility and as an essential determinant of modern active citizenship.

Is it safe?

It could be argued that the experiments in developing a primary care led health service through the 1990s were merely 'tinkering around the edges' in that they did not fundamentally shift the balance of power between primary and secondary care. More recent changes following the government's white papers, *The New NHS: modern, dependable*,[3] and *Shifting the Balance of Power*[4] have placed considerably more responsibility on the primary care sector. One of the constraining forces has been the lack of corporacy and the fear that it would not be safe to trust the primary care sector with power and control of resources.

Figure 10.1 illustrates the kind of balance sheet which observers have to consider when deciding whether it is safe to trust the primary care sector. Each of the elements in this diagram has been discussed elsewhere – except perhaps the threat of the 'poisoned chalice'. This describes the feeling of those accepting power within the primary care sector, who remain unsure whether they are going to be left to hold their new responsibilities without support – to be left holding the baby when the music stops. If the system does not trust PCT organisations sufficiently then direct management by SHAs, increased central control, targets and directives will follow and the chance of building a welfare service based on

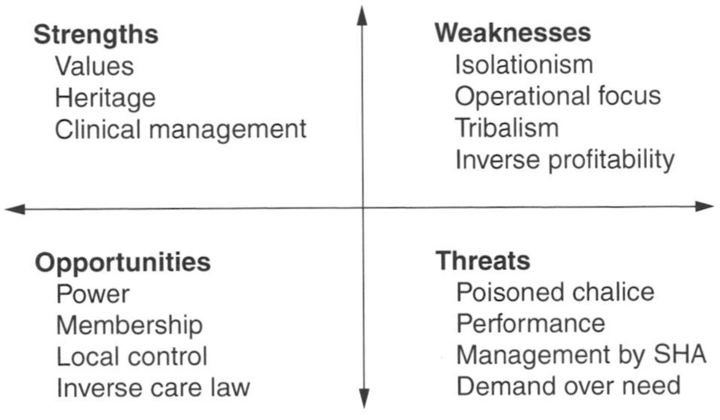

Strengths	Weaknesses
Values	Isolationism
Heritage	Operational focus
Clinical management	Tribalism
	Inverse profitability
Opportunities	**Threats**
Power	Poisoned chalice
Membership	Performance
Local control	Management by SHA
Inverse care law	Demand over need

Figure 10.1:   Primary care – fit for the future?

the needs of local communities will have been lost forever. PCTs will need to demonstrate their maturity and ability to deliver high quality, efficient and effect-ive services very rapidly and in a way that cannot be challenged by the wounded animals in the system such as those who have lost power in the secondary care sector, displaced general managers from health authorities and those who have promoted traditional general practice virtues to maintain the inverse care law and the inverse profitability law.

As demonstrated throughout this book when looking at how systems work, there is always a backwash to introducing change. There is always a risk that the backwash may damage and risk the success of the venture, no matter how well thought out and how carefully planned is the process. Developing corporate organisations in primary care and empowering them to deliver a modern and dependable health service is not a risk-free venture.

Another way of looking at the fitness of primary care for its developing and anticipated responsibilities is to look at the changes in approach and the trends in development that are required. We must balance, in our own minds, the extent to which such development is both consistent with the forces operating on the system and sustainable as those forces evolve and change.

Table 10.3 illustrates four aspects of this issue by looking at the changes in structure, processes, policies and strategies.

Table 10.3:   The future of primary care as a system

Out	*In*
Structure	
National contracts	Community based contracts
Registration	Membership
Professional partnership	Networks
Tribal groups – LMCs, RCGP	Primary care teams
Processes	
Repeat prescribing	Managed therapy
Dispensing	Supply of medicines
Meetings	Organisational consultations
Surgeries	Clinical consultations
Drift	Decisions
Policies	
Uniprofessional	Team
Provider centred	Patient centred
Protectionist	Inclusive
Imposed	Agreed
Strategies	
Widget management	Systems thinking
Gatekeeping	Care co-ordination
Professional paradigms	Community paradigms
Centralism	Peripheralism

Structure

The heritage of the structure in primary care has underpinned the responsibilities of the sector – including registration, expert generalism, independence, gate-keeping and provision of first point of contact care. The heritage of professional partnerships, local representative committees, national contracts and regulations has underpinned and sustained the sector's approach to these responsibilities and by and large these structures have made it possible for the sector to discharge its responsibilities in a way trusted by the community, safe enough for patients and staff to trust with their lives and careers, and sufficiently sensitive to local circumstances. However, as the responsibilities of the sector develop and as the forces operating on the system change so the structures need to adapt. As discussed elsewhere, isolated independent practices and practitioners are now being encouraged to work increasingly in clinical networks across organisations and in teams which span a range of professional paradigms so as to offer patients more cohesive care. Local contracts or agreements between these teams and networks and the PCT or organisation are emerging as a way of encouraging coherence and the promotion of sound governance.

Processes

In adapting the heritage of care provision to the new responsibilities such as some of the processes through which care has been provided and through which the responsibilities of individuals and organisations within the primary care sector have been discharged, it is apparent that the processes cannot be un-affected by change. As has been described elsewhere, the current arrangements for the supply of medicines in primary care owe more to history than to current needs. The repeat prescribing system and the separation between prescribing and dispensing the supply of medicines has been a safe and effective system supporting appropriate treatment for many years. In the world of the Internet, pharmacogenetics and complex specialist care packages being delivered at home, the supply of medicine system is in urgent need not just of evolutionary 'mutation', but of fundamental change. The professionalism of community pharmacists will need to adapt to the 'new managed therapy' paradigm and help general practice out of its fixation on the FP10 and toward a fixation on safe and effective supply of medicines. This is a clear example of the need to move away from looking at the twigs, branches and trees, or the processes and elements making up the system, and towards an approach that looks at the system as a whole, i.e. the wood and the trees, and towards how the system works, its physiology and its dynamics.

Box 10.2:   Polly's pills

Polly is 80 and lives alone in a sheltered flat on the edge of town. She has a number of chronic health problems which require her to be on eight different medicines – some taken once a day, some twice and some three times. In order to ensure that she has the medicines that she requires and takes them at the right times she has a 'medidose' – a container that her daughter fills every week. Polly has to put a written request in to the practice each time that she needs to renew her prescription and has to give them two or three days' notice before the prescription can be picked up. This prescription then needs to be taken to her local community pharmacy for dispensing. Because some of her pills come in packets of 28, some in packets of 30 and some in bottles of 100 they do not all run out together. In the last month Polly has had to order five repeat prescriptions for different items and has had to make 10 trips to the surgery as a result and five trips to the community pharmacy. The practice has now called Polly in for a medicines review, but she will have to wait two or three weeks for this appointment and it will be focused on ensuring that she needs all the medicines she is on and that she is not suffering from any side effects from them, rather than on any attempt to ensure that supplying her with her necessary treatment is as convenient and simple as it could possibly be. Polly has to run her life around ensuring that she is medicated appropriately. She thinks about and checks her medicines every day, and her main topic of conversation and interest in life seems to be her health and her medication rather than her family, friends and the wider world.

Other processes involved in providing care may similarly be in need of review. Traditional consultation patterns involving surgeries and clinics provided at times which suit the organisations and the practitioners may no longer meet modern circumstances. The current problems of access to primary care require opening up the consultation system to new ideas and ways of working to see whether they meet the needs of the community better. Skill substitution, triage, group consultations, involvement of patient interest groups and the voluntary sector, virtual and tele consulting and telephone based follow-up are all approaches which are currently being evaluated.

The way that change has been implemented in primary care over past years has been through a process of gradual evolution rather than planned development. Practitioners and practices have drifted into ways of working and into systems of care, through a process of 'micro-adaptation'. Good ideas have been tried and if they work they have continued and spread throughout the organisation – that is how repeat prescribing has gradually developed. Unfortunately such micro-adaptation is less able to deal with issues requiring more fundamental change. The decision to develop new premises or expand the clinical team or

discipline a bullying employee each requires a different approach. Making decisions in primary care has historically been more through a process of drift, and
achieving a consensus around the status quo, than it has been towards decisive-
ness, openness and responsiveness to changing circumstances. The requirement
in future will be to maintain the sensitivity to local circumstance, and the need
to micro-adapt, so as to ensure that the processes of care are always adapting to
patient needs. At the same time it must be ensured that decisions requiring more
fundamental change are made corporately and are implemented more effectively.

Policies

As illustrated in Table 10.3, the heritage of corporate and clinical policies followed within the primary care sector consists of those that have been appropriate
for a professionally led practitioner centred 'practice' model of care provision.
The policies have not reflected employment practice in other walks of life, e.g.
occupational health and human resource policies. They have not reflected current clinical practice, in providing care through the expertise of a range of professions such as nursing, medicine, pharmacy, occupational therapy, physiotherapy
etc. They have been designed to protect the practitioner's position and the supplicant relationship with patients rather than directed towards improving the
healthcare of the population. They have not encouraged individuals to take
responsibility for their own health. Practices and practitioners have either
imposed policies within their organisations or had them imposed on them by
national or health authority dictate, e.g. NSFs, SAFF agreements, patient protocols
and NICE. They have not seen it as a requirement for policies to be negotiated
with, and agreed with, the parties who are going to be affected by them, such as
staff, patients and their carers and families.

Strategies

As has been discussed when looking at the prescribing system, the focus in primary care has been on 'micro-adaptation' and concentration on every element
of the system rather than on the system 'as a whole'. This approach can be considered as 'widget management' – management of every tiny element of a system
– the twigs rather than the branches, stems and trunks. It makes it very difficult
to see what is going on – to step back and to see the broader picture.

   In future primary care is going to need to take a longer term and more fundamental approach, i.e. to develop some strategic thinking. Thinking long term,
planning and taking a strategic approach to development have not thus far been
characteristics of the primary care sector, but as argued throughout this book
the sector now needs to adopt many of these approaches, which make up the
elements of 'systems thinking'. Leaders in the sector should at least pay some
attention to strategic planning if the sector is to be fit to discharge its responsibilities.

In addition, the heritage of gatekeeping, whereby practitioners have controlled access to external services, will need to respond and adapt to the modern responsibilities of primary care practitioners in terms of co-ordinating care, and ensuring that appropriate care packages are both designed and delivered to meet particular patient needs. This must mean a more fluid approach to delivering care between hospital and home, between home and day centre or residential care and between outpatients and the surgery. Practitioners will need to maintain responsibility for their patient wherever the patient is, rather than feel that once they have referred or delegated care they have discharged their responsibilities. 'Once the rockets are up who cares where they come down, that's not my department' (Werner von Braun as quoted by Tom Lehrer).

With most of the approaches and strategies followed within the primary care sector having historically been based on *professional paradigms* and largely around protecting the power base of medicine, nursing and pharmacy, it is now apparent that a move towards models or paradigms of care which are based on the aspirations of, and developments within, local communities is required. As illustrated in the two futures, Choice First and the Feel Good Factor, these alternative paradigms involve issues about membership and accountability as much as they focus on quality assurance and power sharing. There will always be an inherent tension between and balance required between the requirements of the broader national community as represented by the government, Treasury and national institutions such as CHIA, NICE, NCAA, and the requirements of local communities for approaches which are sensitive to their needs.

This balance between 'centralism' and 'peripheralism' has to feel right for all the parties involved. Right, in the light of all the local and national circumstances and also sufficiently responsive to changes in those circumstances so as to be trusted by the parties.

Modernisation of primary care within the NHS

The forces driving the changes outlined above and in other parts of this book are not confined to the primary care sector or even the NHS or the UK. These are global forces which are affecting the development of mankind at the beginning of the twenty-first century. These are the forces that underpin the development of society and mankind and which influence all aspects of modern life. The consequence of the forces is that the snowball illustrated in Figure 10.2 is rolling down hill, and as a result, the culture in the primary care sector is rapidly changing. Taking Tables 10.4 and 10.5 together we can see how the coherent forces driving change react with the 'backwash' forces resisting change and how the elements involved in the NHS (Table 10.5) and the primary care sector (Table 10.4) are responding.

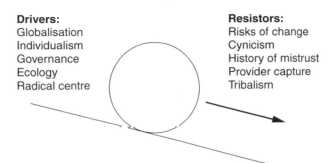

Figure 10.2:   The forces driving primary care.

Table 10.4:   Modernisation of primary care

Forces	Through
Social justice	Membership
Effective care	Quality assurance
Globalisation	Pharmaceutical industry
	Epidemics – HIV
Individualism	Lay majority
	Membership
Governance	Public meetings
	Power sharing
Ecology	Genetics
	Health focus
	Health and fitness
Radical centre	Change through participation
	Responsibility to community and future generations
	Emancipation through knowledge
New dynamics	Membership
	Social inclusion and community spirit
	Synergy of health, housing, social care and environmental planning
	Disengaging local and personal health issues
	From central determination and reliance on economic rather than social forces

The drive of the whole approach is towards promoting social justice for the individuals who make up local, national and world communities. In the health service this drive has led to a focus on community development and targeting issues of social exclusion, such as crime and disorder, lone parenting, substance abuse and discrimination, while in the primary care sector we can anticipate that the response will be towards a membership based organisation, i.e. one which is driven by the needs of its membership and includes the members within its development thinking and accountability systems.

The forces involved in delivering these purposes can also be interpreted in the different areas.

Table 10.5:   Modernisation of the NHS

Forces	Through
Social justice	Membership
Community development	Engagement
Globalisation	Subsidiarity
	Responsibility
Individualism	Active citizenship
	Membership
	PIAs
	Inheritance
Governance	Power sharing
	Limited freedom
Ecology	Sustainability
	Debt to the future
	Holism
Radical centre	Informed choice
	Devolved power
New dynamics	Personal ownership
	Racing on the flat
	Fluid care pathways
	Learning through relationships
	Growing through learning
	Health and contentment

Globalisation

To an ever increasing extent we are all part of one global economy. The pharmaceutical industry markets its products throughout the world and as parallel imports and the supply of effective HIV treatments in southern Africa have shown, no country or PCT can think of itself as an island in these terms. In addition, while we have known for many years that flu epidemics track across the world and influence healthcare in every country, it is now apparent that these forces have caused major transcontinental social and economic development through epidemics such as HIV and foot and mouth disease.

Individualism

The political emancipation of women following the First World War and of men in the eighteenth and nineteenth centuries can be seen as steps upon the path to a broader emancipation of individuals as *citizens*. As they have been offered opportunities in education, become wealthier and live longer without having to devote all their energies to hard labour, so they have been liberated to live more fulfilling lives. The trend to individualism in the NHS can be seen as an element of *'active citizenship'*,[5] while Choice First and the Feel Good Factor point us towards individualism through membership and personal investment accounts. In addition, the rise of genetic medicine can be expected to promote further this approach of individualism. We all inherit our genes from our parents and pass them on to our children. This relationship between the generations and the dependency that each has on that inheritance can be seen as fuelling the rights and responsibilities of every individual. The drive to promote the extent to which individual members of the community are encouraged to take responsibility for their own health is to some extent a response to the criticisms of Ivan Illich.[6]

Developments since Illich published his criticism have largely failed to provide an effective response. The rise of individualism as a social force and in particular the new elements of personal responsibility, membership and genetic health can be expected to grow in importance as a balancing response.

Governance

Across the world the governance of nations and their interdependence is a major source of news every day. Wars, tribalism and dramatic social change such as the destruction of the Berlin Wall and the end of apartheid have shown how the governance of nations can shift relatively swiftly from one paradigm to another. Within the NHS, governance by central control and ministerial dictate has been balanced by the sensitivity of health authorities to more local circumstances. With the balance of power shifting[4] towards a primary care led and determined health service, so the governance of the health service is moving more towards a power sharing model and a model where each organisation has 'limited freedom' to govern itself. The elements of governance considered elsewhere in this book, e.g. power, openness, accountability, probity, responsiveness, etc., are each adapting and will have to continue to adapt to the requirements of modern society. Within the primary care sector the introduction of open public meetings in 1997 marked a radical shift towards a more open and accountable approach. But time has moved rapidly on to the arrangements in PCTs where a Professional Executive Committee (PEC) works with a trust board which has a majority of local lay non-executive members. The balancing or power sharing between the executive committee, the board and the management team is a new type of governing arrangement which can be expected to produce a very different approach to care provision in future. At practice and independent contractor business level we should encourage more open governance arrangements – for example, lay involvement or chairmanship of decision-making boards, annual reports, public meetings and membership.

Ecology

The ecology movement of the 1960s and 1970s[7] served to crystallise thinking around the relationship between the development of modern society and the health of the planet. The issues of sustainable development, e.g. not chopping down all the rain forests, but using wood from forests which are replanted at a rate equivalent to the rate at which the wood is being harvested, has for some years been seen as a middle class foible. Buying food from health shops, vegetarianism, growing your own vegetables and riding bicycles have all been seen as somewhat idiosyncratic and amusing diversions from modern materialism. There are, however, important issues underpinning the need to address the forces of ecology and understanding how the primary care sector and system is developing. Essentially the forces of ecology summarise the debt that we owe to future generations and the requirement to pass on to them a world which is a healthier place for them to live in. The requirement is not to plunder all the resources and to pass on to future generations an ever increasing debt, be it in genetic or economic terms, but to ensure that we as a society leave them a better world than the one we inherited.

Radical centre

While much could be written here about the power of the political force and its instruments, it is worth just restricting ourselves to the effect on the health service. The rise of informed choice, patient power and the devolution of power away from the centre has been instrumental in delivering new corporate primary care organisations. The change of momentum within primary care organisation will come through participation of the members of the local community and through the organisations having an accountability and responsibility relationship to that community and to future generations. The role of emancipation, through access to knowledge and information, as well as through education and training should help individuals grasp the opportunity for more control over their health and their fitness. The merger of health clubs, swimming pools and gymnasiums with health centres and hospitals so that we see health and disease as a continuum and as contributing elements to individual contentment and fairness might be anticipated.

The new dynamic

The dynamics released as a result of these forces are what are driving the snowball down hill (Figure 10.2), as it does the power of the backwash is diffused – the risks of change and cynicism, the history of mistrust and the power of providers and other vested interest groups to dominate the system. As a result, and as illustrated in the two futures, the Feel Good Factor and Choice First, the primary care system is developing its own new dynamic. This dynamic encompasses a balance between central and local control as exemplified by *membership*; a balance between understanding its past and developing its future as exemplified by *learning*; a balance between having a focus on disease management or prevention and focusing on the promotion and maintenance of *health*; a balance between local authority provision and health service provision around the shared elements of environmental *planning*, environmental health, housing and social care; a balance between personal responsibility for health and community responsibility for health; and finally a balance between living for today as opposed to enriching the world for the future. This new dynamic can be illustrated in Figure 10.3 which marks the description of the attributes which a primary care organisation might aspire to.

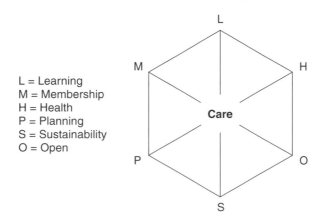

L = Learning
M = Membership
H = Health
P = Planning
S = Sustainability
O = Open

Figure 10.3:   The culture of PCTs.

Each of the adjectives, or elements, describing the PCT in Figure 10.3 is based on the arguments in this book, but perhaps the most important point that Figure 10.3 illustrates is that each of them has to be underpinned by their contribution and relationship to *care* which has been, remains, and must continue to be the heritage of the primary care system.

• A *learning* organisation – one which learns from experience, one which adapts to circumstance, one which invests in its own development and one which develops all its individual members to make its own development sustainable.
• A *membership* organisation – one which is driven by the needs of its members, responds to the views of its members, involves its members in structures and processes and one which is accountable to its members for its performance.
• A *health* organisation as well as a disease management organisation – one which focuses on fitness as well as on care management; one which teaches as well as one which tells.
• *Planning* – an organisation which plans ahead rather than one that simply responds to circumstance; an organisation which consults, involves all stakeholders, reviews its progress and ensures that its activities are coherent with those of its partners.

- *Open* – an organisation whose processes and activities are open to scrutiny; whose structures, committees and subcommittees are inclusive and whose relationships are characterised by high standards of probity and an open and honest approach.
- *Sustainability* – an organisation whose focus and approach is long term; an organisation which builds on the history of biographical care to reflect its responsibilities for future generations and the passing on of a population and a heritage which are fitter. Economic sustainability means balancing the budgets and ensuring that all resources are used wisely, challenging profligacy, but also challenging parsimony and Scrooge-like behaviour where they are damaging to health.

Each of these elements illustrated in the hexagon has to underpin the fundamental heritage of the primary care sector – and in reality of the whole health service – which has to be its focus on *care*. The reason why the NHS represents the best insurance policy that the modern world has seen is that it is based on a contract between every individual citizen and the whole community. The NHS is designed to be there when the individual needs it and he or she contributes to it whenever they are able. The service cares for every individual when they need it and all the organisations, staff and volunteers working with it share the ideal of providing high quality, effective care whenever it is needed. The design of the primary care organisation and system has to focus on that care and its processes, ensuring that all the care it provides is of the highest possible standard.

References

1 Starey N (1996) The primary and community care trust. In: G Meads (ed.) *Future Options for General Practice*. Radcliffe Medical Press, Oxford.
2 Rivett G (1998) *From Cradle to Grave*. King's Fund, London.
3 Department of Health (1997) *The New NHS: modern, dependable*. DoH White Paper, London.
4 Department of Health (2001) *Shifting the Balance of Power: the next steps*. DoH, London.
5 Drucker P (1994) *Post Capitalist Society*. Butterworth-Heinemann, Oxford.
6 Illich I (1976) *Limits to Medicine, Medical Nemesis*. Penguin, London.
7 British Society for Social Responsibility in Science (1970) *Blueprint for Survival*. BSSRS, London.

Index